Sigmund Freud

History of Ideas Series
Paul Roazen, Series Editor

Brother Animal, Paul Roazen
Celebrations, William M. Johnston
Character and Opinion in the United States, George Santayana
Cultural Theory and Psychoanalytic Tradition,
David James Fisher
Doctors and Their Patients, Edward Shorter
Encountering Freud, Paul Roazen
Fathers and Children: Andrew Jackson and the Subjugation of the American Indian, Michael Paul Rogin
Free Associations, Ernest Jones
Freud, Women, and Society, J. O. Wisdom
Helene Deutsch, Paul Roazen
The House of the Prophet, Louis Auchincloss
The Necessity of Choice, Louis Hartz,
edited, compiled, and prepared by Paul Roazen
On the Shoulders of Freud: Freud, Lacan, and the Psychoanalysis of Phallic Ideology, Roberto Speziale-Bagliacca
Oswald Spengler, Stuart H. Hughes
The Psychotherapy of Everyday Life, Peter Lomas
The Public Philosophy, Walter Lippmann
Sexuality, War, and Schizophrenia, Victor Tausk
Sigmund Freud, Helen Walker Puner
Sigmund Freud as a Consultant, Edoardo Weiss
The Therapeutic Process, the Self, and Female Psychology,
Helene Deutsch
Women's Bodies, Edward Shorter

Sigmund Freud

His Life and Mind

Helen Walker Puner

Foreword by Erich Fromm
With a New Introduction by Paul Roazen
and an Afterword by S. P. Puner

Routledge
Taylor & Francis Group
LONDON AND NEW YORK

First published 1947 by Transaction Publishers

Published 2019 by Routledge
2 Park Square, Milton Park, Abingdon, Oxon OX14 4RN
52 Vanderbilt Avenue, New York, NY 10017

First issued in hardback 2019

Routledge is an imprint of the Taylor & Francis Group, an informa business

Library of Congress Catalog Number: 91-44743

Library of Congress Cataloging-in-Publication Data

Puner, Helen W. (Helen Walker), 1915-1989.
Sigmund Freud: his life and mind/Helen Walker Puner; foreword by Erich Fromm; with a new introduction by Paul Roazen and an afterword by S. P. Puner.
p. cm.
Originally published: New York: Howell, Soskin, 1947.
Includes bibliographical references and index.
ISBN 1-56000-611-0
1. Freud, Sigmund, 1856-1939. 2. Psychoanalysts—Austria—Biography. I. Title.
BF109.F74P86 1992
150.19'52—dc20 91-44743
[B] CIP

ISBN 13: 978-1-138-53258-8 (hbk)
ISBN 13: 978-1-56000-611-4 (pbk)

'The public has no claim to learn . . . of my personal affairs—of my struggles, my disappointments and my successes. I have in any case been more open and frank in some of my writings than people usually are who describe their lives for their contemporaries or for posterity. I have had small thanks for it, and from my experience I cannot recommend anyone to follow my example'

—Freud in his Autobiography

'There is a tendency for psychoanalysts to argue that we are entitled to disregard a thinker's opinions when we know enough of his unconscious motives. This point of view invites a *tu quoque.* But I do not propose to ape those bad manners and worse logic by trying to find in Freud's infantile experiences the key to his psychological system.'

—J. L. Grey in Men of Turmoil

'. . . biographers are fixated on their heroes in a very peculiar manner. They frequently select the hero as the object of study, because, for personal reasons of their own emotional life, they had a special affection for him from the first outset. They then devote themselves to a work of idealization, which strives to enroll the great man among their infantile models, and to revive through him, as it were, their infantile conception of the father. For the sake of this wish they wipe out the individual features in his physiognomy; they rub out the traces of his life's struggle with inner and outer resistances, and do not tolerate in him anything savoring of human weakness or imperfection; they then give us a cold, strange, ideal form instead of a man to whom we could feel distantly related. It is to be regretted that they do this, for they thereby sacrifice the truth to an illusion, and for the sake of their infantile phantasies they let slip the opportunity to penetrate into the most attractive secrets of human nature.'

—*Freud in Leonardo da Vinci*

Contents

Introduction to the Transaction Edition

The historiography of psychoanalysis has been an old tale.[1] Although an abundant amount of material has been appearing at an accelerating rate in connection with the story of Freud and his school, certain taboos still remain in place. Just about one hundred years have passed since Freud made public his most distinctive psychological contributions; still, some of the most elementary questions about his life and ideas, as well as the movement he founded, have only now begun to be asked. Freud's name has been so hallowed with religious reverence, and at the same time smeared with villification, that it has been hard for independent observers to evaluate his proper standing in intellectual history.

Looking back on the earliest reception of Freud's work at the turn of the century, some of his critics were capable of being surprisingly perceptive and trenchant.[2] And the first biography ever written of Freud, that by Fritz Wittels in 1924,[3] is still well worth reading today. On the whole, however, most of what has appeared in connection with Freud has been composed for partisan, if not trade-union, purposes. I regret to say that almost all the psychoanalytic journals, however often Freud's name may have appeared in them, have done almost nothing to advance the cause of understanding the early days of psychoanalysis in a way which could approach what one would expect of a proper academic inquiry.

It is in this context that Helen Walker Puner's early book is so outstanding. Its original appearance was one of the reasons that moved Freud's daughter Anna to proceed, against her father's wishes, in authorizing an official biography, which was carried out by Ernest Jones. I do not know how Puner, working in the relative vacuum of knowledge available as of the mid-1940s, could have come up with what she did; but Jones's references to her in volumes 1 and 2 of his biography constitute testimony of his need to counter her influence.

Rereading her book today, I find that Puner's work still stands up and has much to teach, which helps to explain why it has been rarely out of print since its first appearance in 1947. To cite my own initial reaction to her work, her *Freud* was the first place in print that, in the 1960s, I had ever noticed a reference to his being capable of making the diagnostic mistake of calling a physical illness a psychogenic one; and she did so with surefootedness, since she was able to quote Freud himself admitting having committed exactly such an error of thinking a problem was psychological when it turned out not be so at all. Freud was a better critic of himself than many of those could tolerate who afterwards chose to claim his mantle of authority.

Puner was exceptionally sensitive in connection with the important problem of Freud and religious belief. As she put it in writing about Freud's *Totem and Taboo*,

> This view of the religious impulse, which Freud was never to relinquish but only to augment and embroider, left no room for the inclusion of any of the positive elements which have entered into man's need for religion. Freud saw the religious impulse as a purely negative and fear-driven drive, based not on love but on guilt; not on faith but on the need to atone; not on communion with a loved figure but an anxious pacification of a hated figure.

Insights of hers still retain their acuteness; for example, she writes,

> Because Freud wanted to fight against the stern, commanding voice of his father within himself, just as he had wanted to fight the actual voice of his childhood, his conscience, stiffened by opposition, became an unyielding tribunal before which all the less stern, more pleasurable aspects of life were tried and found wanting.

Her Freud was a complex one: "He was a kind, a benevolent, a good man, but he was kind without softness, benevolent without compassion, and good without mercy."

The reader can expect to find extraordinary nuggets of insight from Puner. In order to establish the role of her book in the history of the literature about the creator of psychoanalysis, I would like to quote from a letter she sent me after Kurt R. Eissler, the custodian of Freudian orthodoxy and the founder of the Freud Archives, invited her to dinner in New York City some thirty years after the publication of her *Freud*. The expressiveness of her writing gives an added dimension to her literary capacities, as well as helps to establish the enduring affront to received wisdom about Freud that her book constitutes.

> My dinner at Eissler's house was loathsome—nine courses all covered with cream sauce; clicking of the heels and kissing my hand as he greeted me at his door—looking, it seemed to me, like the rigid, jerky death figure in the Jooss ballet *The Green Table*.
>
> With my last sip of coffee—desperately needed to counteract the *schlagober* [whipped cream] he arose and said it was time for "the debate." I said what debate? But he ignored my remark, and led to his study. I asked, entering, "Is this room bugged?" (In addition to the man's being a lunatic, he has no sense of humor.) He blanched a deeper putty color and mumbled, "Mmm. ha . . . I had thought to tape record this conversation but hmm . . . ah . . . decided not . . ."
>
> He then proceeded to point out to me for about two hours the many "mistakes" I had made in my book. These boiled down to a wrong date and what were, in truth, differences of interpretation, let alone the vast difference of vision that exists when one person is a mensch and the other a whited simulacrum of same. (He is indeed, as I believe you said, an odious combination of

> obsequiousness and grandiosity.) He was particularly exercised over my treatment of Freud as a Jew, and went on for a long time about how happy or well-adjusted Freud was to be a Jew. He also said that geniuses were not human beings—that humans had evolved by adapting to the environment and geniuses stood out against the environment and that therefore Freud wasn't human and I had made a big booboo in treating him as a human being. When I asked him if he found anything valid about my book, he started mumbling again. From what I could make out of the mumble, he was saying that he hears from "professors" here and there with some regularity who write him, "But Helen Puner said this," or "Helen Puner put it this way." I said, "You mean my book is still being taken seriously?" He mumbled sadly, "Very seriously indeed." When I told him I had heard that there was correspondence about my book in the archives, he said loudly, "No." I said my source was informed and reliable. He then said, "I don't know. I get this material all the time and I send it down to the Library of Congress." In other words, he doesn't read it—a liar, the man is also a liar. . . .
>
> The sequel is that he hasn't stopped writing me since I left his house. . . . Basically, he is bombarding me with obsessive material and I am responding with wit and humor—he doesn't know what to make of my answers. . . .
>
> In one of my replies to one of his letters, I thanked him for the rare experience he had afforded me of putting me down while kissing my hand. His reply to this was agitated.

I am citing this letter of Helen Puner's not only for the inherent interest of her encounter with Eissler, who later became celebrated through Janet Malcolm's portrayal of him in connection with Eissler's having hired, and then fired, Jeffrey M. Masson as Projects Director of the Freud

Archives.[4] This quotation also demonstrates Helen Puner's artistic talent and spiritual quality. In writing to me she knew that as objects of Eissler's ire she and I were kindred spirits, since he had, in response to my *Brother Animal: The Story of Freud and Tausk*,[5] launched a polemical attack on my work. In certain orthodox psychoanalytic quarters Eissler is still a "revered" figure;[6] Anna Freud and Eissler were the closest allies right up until her death in 1982. But in the history of those who have tried to approach Freud's life and mind with appreciative detachment, as opposed to worshipful religiosity, Helen Puner's book deserves to be remembered and studied by a new generation of students, who are able to approach his life and struggles without the blinders and prejudices of an earlier time.

Paul Roazen

Notes

1. Paul Roazen, "The Historiography of Psychoanalysis," in *Austrian Studies*, 3, edited by Edward Timms and Ritchie Robertson (Edinburgh: University of Edinburgh Press, 1992).
2. Paul Roazen, Book Review of Kiell, editor, *Freud Without Hindsight: Review of His Work (1893-1939)*, *Journal of the History of the Behavioral Sciences*, January 1990, 197-202.
3. Fritz Wittels, *Sigmund Freud* (N.Y., Dodd, Mead & Co., 1924).
4. Paul Roazen, *Encountering Freud: The Politics and Histories of Psychoanalysis* (New Brunswick, N.J.: Transaction, 1990), pp. 30, 49-51, 76-77.
5. Paul Roazen, *Brother Animal: The Story of Freud and Tausk*, with new Introduction (New Brunswick, N.J.: Transaction, 1990).
6. Paul Roazen, "Letters," *Partisan Review*, 1986, 653-54.

Foreword

It is a pleasure to introduce this biography of Freud. Although it was not written by a professional psychologist, it shows a sensitivity and grasp of Freud's personality and cultural function which is quite unusual. This is all the more remarkable in view of the fact that a biography dealing with the life of a great man always encounters certain difficulties. There are those who idealize the hero and can see in him only the embodiment of all virtue and wisdom. As a consequence, they do not give us the picture of a live man, but the cliché of an idol. The other danger in writing a biography is exactly the opposite. The writer lacks the capacity to admire anybody. He can never see a mountain when he is confronted with it, but reduces everything to plains and little hills. His picture has as little life as that provided by the hero-worshiper.

These difficulties have been most conspicuous in the case of biographies on Freud. He has been less frequently belittled, it is true, although this has been done in many casually printed remarks and articles about him, in which he has been described as an enthusiastic charlatan, or as a representative of a sensuous, decayed Viennese atmosphere. In the formal biographies of Freud it is the danger of hero-worship which has been the most conspicuous. It seems that there are even some psychoanalysts who have not been able to overcome their need to have an idol. They believed themselves free from such infantile impulses as long as they did not worship the current idols in religion or in politics. But they made a religion of psychoanalysis, and an idol of Freud. They saw in him not an unusually creative, imaginative, courageous and uncompromising man, which he was, but a tolerant, kind, just, objective, loving saint, which he was not.

In Freud's case, the unrealistic, sentimental biography is all the more disturbing because it was the very essence of his work to see man realistically; that is, to understand the forces that motivate him and yet of which he is unaware; to recognize that most of what we think about ourselves is well-meant lies, that we are in fact quite different—not necessarily worse—in our real existence, from the legend about ourselves which we create. To make of Freud a legend shows that one has not really absorbed his ideas and discoveries.

Furthermore, one cannot truly approach the analyst, Freud, without seeing connections between his theories and his personality. One has to understand his deep and yet unrecognized attachment to his mother in order to evaluate fully his discovery of the Oedipus Complex. One has to understand his striving to be a world reformer to see that he wanted to conquer the world with an ideal—that of the control of passion by reason—and to understand why Freud built a psychoanalytic movement which was internationally and hierarchically organized.

It is most fortunate that Mrs. Puner's biography of Freud is being published again. Her book is more analytical and realistic than those written by psychologists so far. She looks at Freud with genuine admiration, and yet without idolatry. She understands his own psychological problem and has a full appreciation of the pseudo-religious nature of the movement he created. I am sure that her biography will help greatly to disseminate a true and inspiring picture of the founder of psychoanalysis.

Erich Fromm

Preface

The revolution in man's knowledge of himself as an individual and as a member of society which Sigmund Freud set in motion has only begun to be felt in all its repercussions. Psychoanalysis began at the turn of the century. As a science, it is still in its adolescence. Like all adolescents, it is full of conflict and somewhat unwelcome premonitions of approaching maturity. It cannot at the moment be judged or evaluated finally, for it is still in the process of evolving. For that reason, it should neither be condemned on the basis of the calibre of its individual practitioners nor should it be judged on the basis of any individual factor in the Freudian pattern.

As psychoanalysis develops, any of the specific doctrines which Freud formulated, such as the sexual origin of neurosis or the structure and dynamics of the libido, may be proved to be in error. And it is apparent, from the vantagepoint of nearly half a century, that the weapons which Freud used in his courageous search for universal truth are almost as antiquated as the blunderbuss or the javelin. Yet the Romans conquered a world with little else than an idea and a primitive weapon; and the Spaniards crossed an ocean armed only with faith and the blunderbuss to open a new continent to mankind. In similar fashion Freud, equipped with a faith in reason and an array of scientific ideas now largely outmoded, discovered and explored a new world. Regardless of the areas of that world which may be overthrown in the light of new knowledge, the world itself will persist.

The judgment of posterity is already transmuting his science, which bears the stamp of the era in which it was born, into a trend or method pointing toward evolving knowledge. Since psychoanalysis is already pointing a way for others to pursue, it is a valid and valuable discipline. In proving itself thus far, it has already made Freud, who was so concerned with immortality, immortal.

The man who fathered the ideas which have proven to be so significant for our time was at bottom as fallible and frail as other men. But he worked and moulded the clay which is common to all men into a superhuman structure. This was both his great achievement and his great crime against himself. How and why he did this is the subject of this book. Like any detective fiction which, on the basis of the cumulative circumstantial evidence, uncovers the villain and absolves the hero, this book is an attempt to unravel the mystery of Sigmund Freud's life. Its dénouement, however, is more true of life than it is of fiction. For in the strange case of Sigmund Freud, the villain and hero of the piece are one and the same.

Afterword

Helen Puner was often asked how it came about that she, a journalist, came to write such an upscale book as a biography of Freud. Her answers were modest and uninformative since such questions although often sincere nevertheless carried an overtone that could lead only to her qualifications rather than to substance. Added to all this was the expressed hostility of the Freud family and consequent denial of access to his private papers and family life. She was an "unauthorized" biographer.

But the passage of time has all but buried the pejorative and often caustic criticism (see the "official" Jones biography) and brought to a proper perspective and appreciation the brilliant focus brought by this thirty-two-year-old young woman on probably the most important facet of this many faceted man: the influence of Freud's Jewishness on his professional development. Common understanding these days but remarkably obscure then under the weight of the Master's tonnage of ideas and conclusions.

It came about very simply. In the 1940s in the midst of World War II Helen, then an editor of Fortune Magazine was asked to write a piece on the diagnosis and treatment of "Shell Shock" in World War I and how it had become "Psychoneurosis" in World War II. The piece appeared in 1943 and was called to the attention of the Surgeon General of the United States who promptly had it reprinted and distributed throughout the army medical establishment. How William Soskin, her first publisher, got hold of a copy I do not know but somehow he did. Fresh out of the army and eager to be the first to publish a Freud biography, he got Helen's name from Fortune, called her and proposed the book. She at first refused—the subject being so great—but finally the Gemini in her and the challenge prevailed and although she was a new mother she agreed to do it leaving a maid and a new father to take care of our first born.

Reading deep into the night; interviewing psychiatrists without number as well as rabbis and priests; thinking, mulling and thinking and panicking from time to time, two years later she surfaced with this manuscript. It was quickly published and won a nasty review from an Establishment spokesman: "Journalist!" Happily the last word came from her supporters; "There have been other fragmentary memoirs on Freud but this is the first authoritative and profoundly perceptive biography of the man who more than any other has shaped the thinking of the Western World in this century. It is a brilliant performance, done without fear but doubtless invoking a variety of reproaches."

S.P. Puner

1

Prophecies and Premonitions

Sigmund Freud, whose profound and vigilant mind became the laboratory for psychological discoveries which have shaken the complacent conventions of Western civilization, was born into a world of perplexing reality whose problems he spent a lifetime trying to solve. Perhaps the world which greeted the infant Freud on May 6, 1856, was no stranger than that which has greeted and continues to greet countless other infants. But as he grew older, Sigmund thought it was.

The house in which he was born, at 117 Schlossergasse, in Freiberg, Moravia, a town of some 5,000 Germans and Czechs then a part of the Austro-Hungarian Empire, was commonplace enough. It was a modest, simple, old, two-story house, detached from its neighbours, built of plastered bricks, topped by a slate roof and without ornament. The household into which he was born was not quite so commonplace. Two women looked after him. There was Nanny, old, ugly, acerb, and harsh when the rules of cleanliness were transgressed, but knowing and able. Her wise eyes looked down into the cradle with affection; but the love that shone in the eyes of his mother was so effulgent that it not only lit up the low-ceilinged, close room in which the infant lay, but continued to light the years of his life.

The mother, Amalia Nathanson Freud, was young—

twenty-one when she bore her first child, Sigmund. Slender and pretty, she was the intelligent descendant of a famous Talmudic scholar, the eighteenth-century Nathan Halévy Charmatz of Brody, Poland. The love she radiated for her first-born son was matched only by her vitality. She cooked, she baked, she tended the child; she was alert, sharp-witted and gay. She had borne a child whose destiny it became to make rational the exploration of the irrational and the extra-scientific; but she herself was a believer in signs, portents and premonitions—in all the superstitions of the dark world which begins where reason ends. Sigmund had come into the world covered with a growth of pitch-black hair. His mother interpreted this as a special sign of distinction, and called him in his childhood her "little Moor." She firmly believed and endlessly repeated the prophecy of the old peasant woman who, assisting at the birth, had assured her that she had brought a great man into the world.

This prophecy, a family belief and faith, became a part of the atmosphere in which the child grew up. Later, when Sigmund was a boy of eleven or twelve in Vienna, his mother was to fortify the early legend by interweaving it with a new prophecy. "One evening at a restaurant on the Prater, where my parents were accustomed to take me," Sigmund Freud wrote when he was a man of forty-four, "we noticed a man who was going from table to table and for a small sum improvising verses upon any subject that was given him. I was sent to bring the poet to our table and he showed his gratitude. Before asking for a subject he threw off a few rhymes about myself, and told us if he would trust his inspiration I should probably one day become a 'minister'. I can still distinctly remember the impression produced by this second prophecy. It was in the days of the 'bourgeois Ministry'; my father had recently brought home the portraits of the bourgeois university graduates, Herbst, Giskra, Unger, Berger and others, and we illuminated the house in their honour. There were even Jews among them; so that every diligent Jewish schoolboy carried a ministerial portfolio in his satchel. The impression of that time must be responsible for the fact that until shortly before I went to the university I wanted to study jurisprudence, and changed my mind only at the last moment."[1]

Out of the mother's mystic belief in her first-born's destiny, out of her simple love and pride in him, out of her twice-told tales of the prodigy's progress, she sewed a hero's robe for the child. "Perhaps," one of Freud's sisters once said, "my mother's trust in Sigmund's future destiny played a definite part in the trend given his whole life." Sigmund certainly thought so. Over and over again, in the course of his mature writing, he was to sound this theme: "A man who has been the undisputed favourite of the mother keeps for life the feeling of a conqueror, that confidence of success that frequently induces real success."[2] And when on his seventieth birthday, an occasion of world-wide celebration, he came to review the years he had spent as a child in Freiberg, he found no better way to characterize himself than "the happy child of Freiberg, the first-born son of a youthful mother."

But it was not a simple, unalloyed happiness this child of Freiberg knew. He had an indulgent and admiring mother, but he was also faced with the fact of his father, a man who was forty-one years old when Sigmund was born, virtually twice the age of his wife.

Jacob Freud had owned and operated a small weaving mill against increasing odds. Sigmund's mother was his second wife; and close to the newlyweds' home lived the evidence of Jacob's first marriage—Emmanuel, Jacob's eldest son by that earlier marriage, together with Emmanuel's wife and two children: John, then one year old, and Pauline, a newborn infant.

While it was in no sense extraordinary to become a father again at the age of forty-one, Jacob had the distinction of being a grandfather at the time of Sigmund's birth. Delighted as he may have been at the arrival of a new son in his middle age, he could not have viewed the child with the same rapture as his wife. Babies and sons were an old story to him. His life, more than half over, had been a hard one—a constant struggle to earn a decent livelihood for his family. The losing fight had to a certain extent formed him: he was neither dour nor markedly bitter, but he was stern and jealous of that area of authority he had not succeeded in establishing in the outside world: his authority as a father in the bosom of his family could not be questioned. The traditional Jewish injunction to honour the father must be upheld. Jacob Freud was, none the less, a just man, an intelligent man, one who walked in the faith of his fathers.

But the child, accustomed to the gratification of every wish by an indulgent mother, saw in the father denial, restriction and command. The authority of his father reverberated down the years of Sigmund Freud's life. He brooded over every paternal reproof. He recalled, as a man in middle life, that once when he was an infant barely able to walk he had invaded his parents' bedroom. Driven out by his father's vehement command, he pondered the echo of this denial for a long time, as his recollection of the incident in later life shows.

At the age of two he would still wet his bed. It was his father, not his mother, who reproved him. One of these many reproofs the child remembered all his life. On this occasion he said to his father: "Don't worry, Papa. I will buy you a beautiful new red bed in Neutitschein [the district capital]."

John, the son of Jacob's son, Emmanuel, was Sigmund's closest friend and playmate. In the quarrels which frequently developed between the two children, Jacob would act as judge and hanging jury. "Why did you hit John?" the father would demand. And whether the young Sigmund answered or not, the posing of the question alone seems to have been for him evidence of an unwarranted exercise of authority difficult to absorb in the face of his mother's unquestioning acceptance of him.

The contradiction between Jacob's attitude towards him and Amalia's attitude towards him puzzled the child. But there was a further contradiction, even more difficult to understand. For while his father stood for grim authority, he was oddly also his playmate, a provider of a kind of delight that was to afford for the mature Sigmund Freud inspiration and solace. Jacob would take him, even before he was old enough to walk, into what he always remembered as "the beautiful forest." Freiberg was only a half-mile from a dense forest in the gentle foothills of the Carpathian mountains—then a peaceful pastoral countryside. These walks with his father, which became a regular part of their life together, were times of happiness for the child. They provided a truce in their embattled relationship. Alone together in the quiet of the woods, the father would seem to the child not the care-worn, middle-aged man who addressed him with the forbidding voice of authority, but a gentle companion. The forest itself, with its constant change and renewal, was a place of wonder. It became in a sense a home of the heart for the child to which he continued to resort, and in which he found renewal all his life.

Despite his instinctive recoil from and unconscious rebellion at the stern voice of parental authority, Sigmund came to regard his father (as most children do!) as the wisest, most powerful and wealthiest man in the world. In fact, Jacob Freud was by virtue of his patriarchal position, and by the aura of authority which he imposed, the summit of the hierarchy of family authorities. First to be feared in Sigmund's eyes was Father. Next came Emmanuel, that equivocal figure who was at once his own half-brother and the father of his contemporary, John. Then Nanny, who was as often forbidding as she was kind and affectionate. Then John, the Janus-faced nephew who, by reason of his slightly greater age and strength, could oppress Sigmund as readily as he could co-operate with him. Last, Mother, who rarely exerted any arbitrary authority at all.

The family hierarchy confused the child not only because so many people were in positions of authority over him, but because of the virtually incomprehensible relationship of the people who constituted it The sharp eyes with which he had been born, lustrous, brown and scrutinizing, puzzled over the family constellation, sought an answer beyond the understanding of a three-year-old. He found, of course, no satisfactory solution, but his eyes and mind grew sharper in the search.

There was his mother, young and pretty. She looked, acted and was in fact a contemporary of his father's sons by his first marriage, Emmanuel and Philip, and Emmanuel's wife. Jacob, Sigmund's father, was closer to Nanny's age and outlook than he was to Amalia's. The evidence of his eyes told the child that by all laws of congruity, Jacob should be married to Nanny and Amalia to Emmanuel. Jacob, his father, was the grandfather of John, his playmate. His own relationship to his father in point of time as well as of family configuration was more nearly that of a grandson than a son. Sons were grown-up men, like Emmanuel.

In his earliest dreams and the childhood fantasies he recorded in later life, the child attempted to reconcile this fantastic world of incongruous realities with one more reasonable and easier to grasp. Sigmund was just two and a half years old when his mother gave birth to another child, Anna. Sigmund was not amused. Here was another riddle: How and why had this little usurper been born? Were more and more little sisters, in engulfing succession, to make their appearance and deflect the warm stream of his mother's love for him? There was another puzzling circumstance to contend with. Immediately after his sister was born, Nanny disappeared. Two riddles then: where had Anna come from? where had Nanny gone to? Although this concern for solving ultimate riddles might seem precocious in a two-and-a-half-year-old, Freud in later life recalled that he had at the time found an answer. Emmanuel—for Sigmund sensed that it was he who had played a decisive rôle in Nanny's disappearance—had made Nanny vanish. (Nanny had been caught stealing, and it was Emmanuel who had her jailed.) And, he concluded, it was the same culprit, Emmanuel, who had slipped the baby inside mother.

In other dreams and fantasies of his early childhood, the boy substituted Emmanuel for Jacob. Emmanuel, not Jacob, was the father, the voice of fantasy said, reasonably enough. The child needed to find a substitute to take on the heavy burden of hostile emotion he bore for his father. If, the wish behind the fantasy said, Emmanuel and not

Jacob was the father, terrifying, omniscient, the creator of the mother's child, then there would be no necessity to be torn between love and fear of Jacob. Jacob, the wish said, could then be loved as wholeheartedly as Amalia.

The wish was not father to the fact. The child's feeling for Jacob remained divided. His relationship to his father and to the family circle grew more paradoxical as he grew old enough to attempt to unwind the tangled skein. Young "Sigi" was the eldest son of his parents, but at the same time, he was the youngest son in the augmented family circle. He was for the first two and a half years of his life the only child of Jacob and Amalia; yet he had two elder half-brothers, Emmanuel and Philip, and for all practical purposes, a young brother and sister, John and Pauline, the children of Emmanuel. To compound the confusion, these brother and sister equivalents were in reality his nephew, one year older than himself, and his niece, roughly his own age. So his position in the family was full of uncertainty. He was an eldest and an only son with all the privileges of his uniqueness. At the same time he was junior to his nephew—the younger of two children brought up as inseparable companions with all the drawbacks inherent in that relationship. An uncle in name only, his equality with John was in John's eyes always debatable. And so was the whole question of his relation to John—for John, his playmate and his contemporary, called Sigmund's father "grandfather."

In a sense, young Sigi's life with John reproduced in miniature the emotional colour of his relationship to his father. First, he must have felt as uncertain of the nature of the blood tie which linked him to John as he was of the nature of the one which linked him to his father. John, he was told, was his nephew. But by virtue of his seniority and strength, by virtue of all the evidence with which Sigi's eyes presented him, John should have been the uncle and he the nephew. John and he were brought up as brothers. But John was no brother; he was the child of a brother. Second, while John was a dearly loved comrade, he was also a threatening rival. John loved Sigi, but in the immemorial manner common to children of all ages and societies, he beat him up when he had the chance.

Thus John came eventually to symbolize to the bewildered Sigi the same mixture of conflicting emotions—of love against fear, friendship against enmity, equality against authority—that he felt for his father.

The two children were inseparable companions. They loved each other and fought each other. They were one day David and Jonathan, and the next day Caesar and Brutus. John was frequently a tyrant who took advantage of his greater age and strength to bully his young uncle. But Sigi, young as he was, was bent on warding off permanent submission. He fought back, despite the unequal odds and despite the love he felt for John.

When, as a man, Sigmund Freud came to review his childhood, he said over and over again that his ambivalent relationship with John had conditioned the course of his character. He never tired of emphasizing and re-emphasizing this point in the pages of *The Interpretation of Dreams*. In speaking of his boyhood hero, Hannibal, he said: "And perhaps the development of this martial ideal may be traced yet father back, to the first three years of my childhood, to wishes which my alternately friendly and hostile relations with a boy a year older than myself must have evoked in the weaker of the two playmates."

Then, speaking of a dream in which Brutus and Caesar appeared, he said: "Strangely enough, I once did play the part of Brutus. When I was a boy of fourteen, I presented the scene between Brutus and Caesar in Schiller's poem to an audience of children, with the assistance of my nephew, who was a year older than I, and who had come to us from England. . . . Until the end of my third year we had been inseparable; we had loved each other and fought each other, and, as I have already hinted, this childish relation has determined all my later feelings in my intercourse with persons my own age. My nephew John has since then had many incarnations, which have revivified first one and then another aspect of a character that is ineradicably fixed in my unconscious memory. At times he must have treated me very badly, and I must have opposed my tyrant courageously. . . ."[3]

Again: "My present . . . annoyance . . . draws reinforcements from springs that flow far beneath the surface, and so swells to a stream of hostile impulses towards persons who are in reality dear to me. The source which furnishes the reinforcement is to be found in my childhood. I have already said that my warm friendships as well as my enmities with persons of my own age go back to my childish relations to my nephew who was a year older than I. In these he had the upper hand, and I early learned how to defend myself; we lived together, were inseparable and loved one another, but at times, as the statements of other persons testify, we used to squabble and accuse one another. In a certain sense, all my friends are incarnations of the first figure; they are all *revenants.* My nephew himself returned when a young man, and then we were like Caesar and Brutus. An intimate friend and a hated enemy have always been indispensable to my emotional life. I have always been able to create them anew, and not infrequently my childish ideal has been so closely approached that friend and enemy have coincided in the same person; but not simultaneously, of course, nor in constant alternation, as was the case in my early childhood."[4]

But there can be little doubt that all this discussion of John, a playmate who was after all not so different from many other playmates who have tormented countless other little boys, screens the memory of the man in whom Sigmund first encountered the bitter brew of divided love—his father. Even as a man, Sigmund Freud could not bring himself to desecrate his father's memory by admitting that the love he bore him was something less than wholehearted.

Beyond the oddly augmented family circle which was the immediately perceived world of the child, stretched the larger, more dimly perceived world of the town and the country.

Freiberg was a peaceful little town with a beautiful name—Free Mountain—about one hundred and fifty miles north-east of Vienna. Pastoral, sleepy, it clung to a steep bank over the Lubina River, a little trickle in summer, but swollen and broad in spring. Dominating the town was the steeple of St. Mary's Birth Church, which stood more than two hundred feet high and had the best chimes in the province. Around the large square in the centre of the town stood arcades of substantial houses, one of them decorated conspicuously with a memorial of the Thirty Years War—a coat of arms, granted "For Valour." It displayed on a field of gold and red two big, vicious-looking pruning knives. In those glorious days, the Freiberg citizenry had distinguished themselves for their endurance, toughness and belligerence. "Brieg, Freiberg and Bruenn make Swedish arms thin," ran the local proverb. Off the market-place, with its religious and martial reminders, its steeple and its pruning knives, close to fields and pastures, lived the Freud family.

It was not by chance that the steeple of St. Mary's dominated the town of Freiberg. Fully ninety-five per cent of the Moravian population was Roman Catholic. Less than three per cent was Protestant, and only two per cent were Jews. Since 1851, Austria had been governed by the political reaction of the Restoration which had been set off by the short-lived liberal revolution of 1848. This return to a darker era did not directly affect people who kept away from politics as the Freud family did—even though Jacob and Emmanuel had been deeply impressed by the short resurgence of freedom which had existed between 1848 and 1851. However, the ill-fated revolution had touched off a situation from which it was less easy to withdraw. It had established Czech nationalism as a moving force in Austrian politics and had thus strengthened the hatred of the Czechs for the Germans, the ruling class in Moravia. The Jews, who in language and education were German, thus became the objects of Czech anti-Semitism.

As a young man in Freiberg, Jacob had felt the brunt of German anti-Semitism, but, as Jews have for centuries, he had borne it resignedly, knowing it to be the inevitable heritage of Jewish birth. And it had been relatively easy to bear because of the comparative Moravian freedom from restrictions. But when the revolution of 1848 hit Bohemia, neighbour of Moravia, it started with Czech riots in Prague directed against Jewish textile manufacturers. Hostility from both Germans and Czechs threatened the Jews, and even in tiny Freiberg, the aroused cloth-makers began to hold the Jewish textile merchants responsible for their plight.

Although the lives and property of the few Jewish families in Freiberg were not actually in danger, the future looked ominous.

The industrial revolution was succeeding where the political one had failed. Everywhere in Central Europe machines were replacing handwork. Even peaceful little Freiberg was locked in its death struggle with the machine, and the traditional method of cloth manufacture which was Freiberg's main source of income, as well as Jacob Freud's, had been steadily declining since 1835. In the 'forties, the new Northern Railway linking Vienna to Germany and Galicia had bypassed the tiny handicraft town, dooming it to slow economic death and increasing unemployment among its artisans. In 1852 a serious inflation began to accelerate the death throes, and by 1859, when Sigmund Freud was three years old and the Austro-Italian war broke out, the town was drawing its last economic breath.

Nothing remained in Freiberg to compensate the Freuds for their loss of dignity and livelihood. The educational opportunities which Freiberg had to offer a bright boy were virtually non-existent. It is true that two years after Sigmund was born, the gymnasium (high school), which had been closed since 1827, was partially reopened. The reopening was made possible by a fund which over a period of thirty years had at last grown sufficiently to permit the establishment of the lowest grades. But with the town's economy expiring, it did not appear likely that full educational facilities would ever develop.

Want of freedom, want of bread and economic opportunity have always been the motives for migration—as much in the nineteenth century as in the twentieth. Jacob Freud's ancestors had been on the march for centuries.

(As his son once wrote: "I have reason to believe that my father's family were settled for a long time on the Rhine at Cologne; that as a result of a persecution of the Jews during the fourteenth or fifteenth century, they fled eastwards, and that in the course of the nineteenth century they migrated back from Lithuania, through Galicia into German Austria.") So in 1859, the Freud family's enforced migration was resumed, as it was to be resumed again some eighty years later. Emmanuel with his wife and two children went to Manchester, where it was hoped that his experience with cloth would stand him in good stead. Jacob with his wife and two children started on a journey to a big foreign city—Leipzig. After a long ride in a horse and wagon, Sigmund got his first sight of a railroad. And after a train ride of many hours, he found himself permanently bereft of his beloved home, of the "beautiful forest," the rolling hills, the tall imposing spire of St. Mary's, of Emmanuel and John.

The train whisked Sigmund Freud from the scenes of his early childhood and from the memory of it. In middle life, he recalled hardly an episode from the year the family spent in Leipzig and from the two or three years following their removal to Vienna. All he remembered was that "those were hard times, not worthy to be recalled."

These are the memories which Freud retained of the first three years of his life. He was a first-born son, warm and wanted in the love of his young mother, secure in her admiration. But he was not his ageing father's first-born, and he encountered in his father a love tempered with justice and age, undemonstrative in comparison to his mother's, and mixed with considerations of morality and righteousness. The child's attitude towards his mother was simple and direct: he loved her wholeheartedly. For his father he felt, even in these first three years of his life, that irreconcilable blend of love and fear that was to determine much of the way he lived his life.

This emotional world was already established in his "happy years" in Freiberg. And so was the strange, now friendly, now hostile, world of reality. From Freiberg, the place of the free mountains, his father had been cast out.

His father, the dispenser of justice and the arbiter of morals, had been defeated by a machine and by the high steeple in the market-place which housed a music that Sigmund Freud was thereafter to avoid. His God, his father's God, was not the God of the market-place. If the child did not understand the reasons for the exodus, he understood well enough the necessity to question it.

He understood, too, or felt compelled to question the family relationships he found within his own household. This child who as a man was concerned with incest, with sexuality, and with the content of what he was derisively accused of establishing as "the family romance," found, within the oddly contorted pattern of his own family, seed enough for his later concern. The world of reality is difficult enough for a child to grasp. But when that world is a place where fantasy is more rational than fact, where semblance is more congruent than reality, the child, to establish his bearings, must question. He must, as the inclination was born in Sigmund Freud in the first years of his life, examine each separate phenomenon. He is likely to feel that the world ruled by tradition-bound authority is suspect.

It would be absurd to assert—even with all due respect to the science Sigmund Freud was later to develop—that his character was completely formed in the first three years of his life in Freiberg. What *was* formed was the predisposition to penetrate and dissect the world of "reality"; to resist the dictates of authority; to find in an object of love, as he had found in his father and in John, an identical object of hate; to be convinced, not so much reasonably as emotionally, of the greatness of his destiny.

2

The New Home

Vienna, the "Queen of German Cities," to which Sigmund Freud moved as a child of four, was enough of a melting-pot then to absorb a few more Jews. There Teuton, Slav and Magyar met, and newspapers were published in German, Hungarian, Polish, Ruthenian, Czech, Slovak, Serbo-Croatian, Slovene, Rumanian and Italian. Mozart had lived there, distilled his spirit into a sunny musical essence, and there his body had been thrown into an unmarked grave in a potter's field. There Franz Schubert had also lived, composed and nearly starved. And Haydn had come to Vienna as a boy, to compose the Masses which "praise God with a cheerful heart."

Vienna was musical, Vienna was gay, Vienna had transformed *gemuetlichkeit*—the condition of being comfortable—into an art form. But the famous Viennese *gemuetlichkeit*, with its graces and its gaiety, its abandon, wit and glitter, constituted only the icing of the baroque cake that was the real city. The palatable icing concealed the fact that the cake sagged sadly, that it was made partly of ersatz flour, and that it contained a few putrescent plums.

For *gemuetlichkeit*, art form though it might be, was also the quintessence of self-indulgence. The Viennese, like some collective *grande dame*, held their skirts apprehensively clear of the mud of sharp convictions, harsh conflict, concentrated effort, and the more sober virtues which characterized the citizens of their Teutonic sister-cities.

The hypocrisy inherent in the political and social scene of the time fortified the natural Viennese inclination to shrug a graceful shoulder and turn the other way when unpleasant facts had to be faced. Austria was a monarchy, constitutional in name only. The constitutional paraphernalia—a parliament of two houses, a charter of rights and liberties, independent law-courts, ministers—were all there. But the real governmental power was vested in the hands of the topmost top of the Austrian aristocracy, an aristocracy which had married and intermarried among themselves with such monotony that it had become a homogeneous whole—one big, happy, dissolute family.

At the head of the family sat the last of the Hapsburgs, the Emperor Franz Josef, who had been reigning for twelve years when little Sigmund arrived in Vienna. Conservative, stubborn, devoted to detail and devoid of vision, he was completely cut off from the life of the people by the fantastically formal court etiquette and by the band of aristocrats who also doubled as court functionaries. This aristocracy was graceful, complacent and callous. Its influence acted as a brake on all initiative in public life. The weight of amorphous, irresponsible power the aristocrats wielded was enough to stifle any innovation and discourage any new forces from attempting to combat them. Although they considered themselves "conservatives," their effect was as feudal as the era from which they derived their power.

Most Viennese chose to ignore the wide gap between apparent democracy and genuine autocracy, for the gap was symptomatic of the cleavage between form and content which pervaded the whole of Viennese life. To arrive at any position of eminence in this society, one required sponsorship from "above." If the aspirant had no direct entrée into the ruling world, it was still possible to lay his case before one of the henchmen to whom the rulers had delegated their power. Without either of these preliminary gambits, no venture could come to fruition; with them, almost any law could be transgressed.

In such a society, the highest social aim was to appear to be a member of the aristocracy, and the middle class, with the rich Jews leading the pack, proceeded to imitate its model down to the last flourish and intonation. The result resembled the glitter and tone of the second act finale of a Lehar operetta, with all the sweet seduction and charm of melody and all the hollowness and inanity of words and action.

Even physically, Vienna was a musical comedy hodgepodge with the scene shifting rapidly from the noble prince's palace to the humble heroine's simple slum. Vienna, by the end of the nineteenth century, had acquired a physicial aspect which aptly expressed its preference for decoration and ornament over function. Beautiful baroque palaces—notably Prince Eugen's—and splendid Gothic cathedrals rose in the midst of dreary streets and humdrum suburbs. Some visitors saw none of the squalor and remembered only the splendour. As one well-pleased observer put it, Viennese architecture was "a happy blending of South German kindliness with Hungarian fire, Bohemian idiosyncracy and Italian intellect and imagination." And by the city, of course, flowed the great and romantic river, the noble and picturesque river, the Danube, suggesting to the Viennese, as this same observer felt, "that the true value of life is to glide with beauty, dignity and grace down the unintelligible river of existence."[5]

Glide or waltz, the true Viennese was mainly concerned with the impression he was creating. He would spend money freely to maintain his own illusion that he was as aristocratic a fellow as the next one. This tendency culminated in the Viennese tradition of *trinkgeld*—giving and receiving tips. Tips flowed as freely in Vienna as the champagne did at Sacher's. As Hanns Sachs says, "Every door you had to pass was opened for you by someone who demanded a tip; you could not get into the house in which you lived after 10 p.m., nor seat yourself in the car in which you wanted to ride without giving a tip. Karl Kraus, Vienna's witty satirist, said that the first thing a Viennese would see on the day of Resurrection would be the outstretched hand of the man who opened the door of his coffin."[6] Dining in one of the better restaurants, the Viennese was expected to give four different tips—one for the head waiter, one for the waiter who served the food, a third for the waiter who served the drinks, and the last for the "Piccolo", a junior waiter-in-training who either helped with the customer's coat, or just hovered. In return for this liberal shower of required gratuities, the waiter was careful to address the diner by the title just above the one to which he was entitled. Thus, Sachs, in the coffee house he frequented, was addressed as "Herr Doktor" as long as he was a student. Upon the day of his graduation he moved up to "Herr von Sachs"—equivalent to the French "Monsieur de." He never, however, made the top rung, which was "Herr Baron."

All Vienna loved this sort of play-acting. All Vienna was stage-struck, and discussions of the theatre, of plays and actors easily took precedence over all other more significant matters of the public concern.

The famous politeness and amiability of the Viennese was part of this game. "To believe," Hanns Sachs says, "that any real result would come of a smoothly played scene would have been as naïve as to expect that an actor would continue in the character of his part after the fall of the curtain. Not only the shopkeeper in his store, but even the high dignitary in his office assured the visitor . . . that he was quite overwhelmed by so much kindness and condescension; but when the scene had been acted, it was all over and nothing came of it. On the other hand, two people who had quarrelled violently became friendly again like a pair of actors who had insulted each other in a dramatic scene."[7]

In the first half of the nineteenth century, when Metternich was Chancellor, Vienna had been the nerve centre of European politics. There the Congress of Vienna had met in 1815 to settle the fate of a continent. Even then, however, the Viennese were more interested in eating and drinking, in burlesque and banter, than they were in liberty, equality and fraternity. A wit of the time cast his cynical eye over the proceedings, and summed them up: *Le Congrès danse, mais ne marche pas.*

By the turn of the century Jews constituted ten per cent of Vienna's population. When the Freud family arrived, they were not as conspicuous in Vienna as they had been in Freiberg by reason of their Jewishness. There was nevertheless more discrimination against Jews in Vienna than there had ever been in the place of the Free Mountain.

Vienna had always had a "Jewish question" because it had for many centuries, since the early days of the Roman Empire, had Jews. When Rudolph, the first Hapsburg, took over, there were so many Jews in Vienna that an Ecclesiastical Christian Synod decreed that they must all distinguish themselves from Christians by wearing a special sort of hat. Forty years later, the hat having become unfashionable, the Jews were introduced to a new style of distinction. They were confined to a ghetto in the northwestern section of the city. The ghetto gradually evolved into a city within a city, with its own schools, park, hospital, taverns, bath-houses and graveyard.

Then, in the late fourteenth and early fifteenth centuries, a series of three pogroms took place which all but wiped out the Viennese Jews. All their property was confiscated, their synagogues torn down—the stones of the synagogues were used to build the University—their houses sold, and their graveyards allotted to Christians.

Two centuries later, however, the Emperor found that Jews could be useful as tax-collectors, and set aside a part of the city (now the Leopoldstadt) for a new ghetto. In 1670, the tide of good will ebbed and the Jews were again expelled from Vienna and their synagogues converted into churches. In the next century, as one Jewish historian has put it, "Maria Theresa disliked them very much." In spite of this dislike, it soon became evident that Austrian commerce was suffering from the absence of Jews, and again in the reign of the "enlightened" Joseph II the Jews were allowed to return to active life. They were permitted to learn handicrafts, to study the arts and sciences, and to farm if they obeyed certain restrictions. They could even attend universities. Joseph abolished the body tax they had been required to pay, and decreed that they need no longer wear beards or stay indoors on Sunday mornings and holidays. The Jews, however, did not receive full citizenship or complete freedom of worship or residence in Vienna. They did get a Magna Charta of sorts: the Emperor decreed in 1781 that they were fellow-men and that Christians should be good neighbours to them. But the era of good-fellowship was again short-lived; soon the old dislike prevailed once more and the old discriminations were gradually restored. By the time the Congress of Vienna, which took a very gloomy view indeed of innovations and improvement, was held in 1815, the Viennese Jews were little better off than they had been in the Middle Ages.

Finally, by 1867, when Sigmund Freud was a boy of eleven and had been living in Vienna for seven years, the Jews were granted in the new constitution equal status with all citizens. Although the constitution put a legal end to racial discrimination, Vienna continued during the rest of the century in which Freud grew to manhood (and afterwards, of course) to remain a distinctly anti-Semitic city.

While the Jews began to dominate the professional, artistic and intellectual life of Vienna, the hurdles and handicaps they had first to overcome remained formidable.* They were looked upon as aliens; they were snubbed and humiliated; they were considered essentially unassimilable—despite the overwhelming concern of the rich Jews to assimilate themselves as rapidly and unobtrusively as possible.

Jacob Wassermann, who came to Vienna in 1898, after having lived in Germany, saw and mercilessly described the effect this was having on the ascendant but unhappy Jews themselves: "One circumstance puzzled me before I had long been in Vienna. In Germany I had associated with Jews scarcely at all; . . . here, however, it developed that all with whom I came into intellectual or friendly contact were Jews. The banks, the press, the theatre, literature, social organizations, all lay in the hands of the Jews.

* By the turn of the century, the overwhelming majority of Viennese lawyers were Jewish, as was a large percentage of the doctors. In one hospital, for instance, twenty-three out of the twenty-four doctors were Jewish.

The explanation was easy to find. The aristocracy would have nothing to do with such things; with the exception of a few who saw things in a different light, they not only maintained a respectful distance from intellectual and artistic life, but feared and condemned it. The small number of untitled patrician families imitated the aristocracy; the original upper middle class had disappeared, leaving a gap now occupied by government functionaries, army officers and professors; then came the closed circle of the lower middle class. The Court, the lower middle class, and the Jews gave the city its stamp. And that the Jews, as the most mobile group, kept all the others in continuous motion is, on the whole, not surprising.

"Yet I was amazed at the hosts of Jewish physicians, attorneys, clubmen, snobs, dandies, proletarians, actors, newspapermen and poets. . . . The German Jews among whom I lived had accustomed me to more polished manners, a less conspicuous demeanour. Here I could never lose a certain sense of shame. I was ashamed of their conduct and their bearing. . . ."

Wassermann, a man who had come from a country where the Jews had achieved their greatest triumph of assimilation, and who could therefore remain comfortably oblivious of the centuries of persecution his co-religionists had suffered, felt that the Viennese Jew's conduct was characterized by a "mistrust that betrayed the Ghetto left not far behind; [*by*] unshakable opinions; idle meditations upon simple matters; sophisticated fencing with words where a seeing eye would have sufficed; servility when pride would have been proper; boastful self-assertion when modesty was in place; lack of dignity; lack of restraint; lack of metaphysical aptitude. . . .

"Through all these Jews ran a duality of rationalism. . . . Among the base it found base expression in worship of success and wealth, in self-seeking and lust for gain. . . . Among the nobler it manifested itself in impotence in the ideal and intuitive realms. Science was set up as an idol, intellect as the sovereign lord. Whatever could not be calculated was relegated to a lower category. Even destiny became a matter of calculation, and the most obscure secret depths of the soul were subjected to a minute analysis."[8]

Leaving aside all considerations of cause and effect, the fact remains that the Jews of Vienna were a group set aside and rejected by the other ninety per cent of the population. They might work in the professions and the arts side by side with Gentiles, but they were not a part of them.

Whatever indictment one may find of Vienna's prejudice, her hypocrisy, her lassitude and her lack of high purpose, the pretty city had one important, counterbalancing virtue, and that was her vitality. Vienna was gloriously alive. And for the young Jew growing up in its midst, the city had a further virtue—it was dynamic with the ferment of new rationalist values and ideas that were the product of the industrial revolution. That revolution which had been sweeping aside the old order in England and France for a hundred years came late to Central Europe. The new social and economic order it created hit Vienna suddenly and violently, and its impact produced psychological changes of a radical nature. Vienna's professional and commercial classes, increasingly Jewish as the industrial revolution progressed, were forced to an eminently rational defense of the new ideas.

For the Jews, newly liberated physically from the ghetto, and liberated emotionally from the faith of their fathers as the world about them opened up, "the dead weight of finality" was gone. They showed, as Wassermann had observed, a reverence for the new rationalist, mechanistic values. Science, which had set them free, was indeed their idol. Intellect, which was the instrument which would keep them free, was indeed the sovereign lord of the day. The same precision that went into the construction of a machine tool was the process which men of science began to take over as the new, infallible weapon in the search for truth.

Growing up in the midst of this old world riddled piercingly and suddenly by the new, a boy like Sigmund Freud could not fail to be influenced by the striking duality of the forces that shaped the life about him. As a Jew, he synthesized in his person the new in the old. As a personality already inclined to withstand the onslaughts of authority, whether parental or social, he would naturally be attracted to the new scientific method which exalted mechanism and rationalism over the traditional ways of faith and mysticism. Nor could the boy, struggle as he might to pay exclusive allegiance to the new, shake off the influence of the old. Not only was Vienna, despite its surface gaiety, in a sense a battlefield upon which the old struggled with the new, but the boy himself had inherited the spirit and the atmosphere of an ancient Judaic tradition. This struggle, this conflict between two opposing forces, was to be reflected in the structure of his character and his work. A profound dualism always distinguished his psychoanalytic theories.

Impressed as he was by the social conflict inherent in Viennese society, his predisposition to penetrate beneath the surface of things must have been fortified by the contrast between Vienna's gay outer existence and the reality of her rigid, Catholic inner life. He found, this boy whose eyes had already been turned towards inquiry by the disparity between the semblance and reality of his own family relationships, the same duality of semblance and reality in the society about him. Under the *Schlagober* in the café, there was the Cross that marked the church, just as under the surface harmony that marked his family there was the suggestion of a dark, irrational but eminently desirable order that contradicted the validity of the reality he saw about him.

Nor could he fail to be impressed, as a Jew, by the disrepute in which the Viennese held the Jews. He saw all about him the eagerness with which the richer Jews rushed to identify themselves with the society which scorned them. He became, as he was subjected to anti-Semitism in school, as scornful of the turncoats who sought to appease their oppressors by becoming indistinguishable from them, as he was of the oppressors themselves. The independence and pride that had been born in him, coupled with the conviction of his destiny that his mother had fostered in him, held him firmly away from the path of assimilation, attractive as that path might appear.

The contrast, then, between the style in which Vienna lived—the gay, formal waltz she stepped—and the content of that life, as full of dark social and religious imponderables as any symphony which Beethoven composed there, was a further incentive to the boy's inquiring mind to probe beneath the semblance in search of the reality. For the semblance, young Freud quickly developed a scorn. The great gregariousness and sociability of the Viennese people he abjured. Music, which was Vienna's spiritual bread, gave him no pleasure. For the glitter, the social graces and the play-acting he felt a tired tolerance.

But he was, nevertheless, marked in certain ways by the city that afforded him the same two-edged sanctuary it afforded other Jews. Freud grew to manhood with a typical Viennese urbanity. He never forgot when a present was due, or where a visit or kind word might bring happiness to a friend. His ironical wariness was also typically Viennese, as was his love for the Viennese card game of *tarock*. His wit and love for pointed stories, which was at bottom Jewish, was related, too, to the *wienisch* love for exaggerated, melancholy irony. And the way he wrote and the way he expressed himself reflected to a certain extent the uneasy marriage of the two cultures in which he found himself, Jewish and Viennese.

The influence of his Viennese upbringing on Sigmund Freud is important to understand because it has been so misrepresented. When Freud's theories first began to attract world-wide notice, and when a shocked world's instinctive reaction to the thesis that sexual maladjustment was the root of neurosis was to mock and condemn its author—the charge that only sensuous, dissolute, degenerate Vienna could have produced such a monstrous travesty of science gained wide circulation. This charge itself is a travesty of the truth. Vienna confirmed the suspicion that had already been born in him, that all was not on the surface what it appeared to be. And, in continuing to treat

him as a suspect Jewish alien in the midst of a seemingly warm and seemingly joyous atmosphere, it hardened his resolution to stand free and independent of the world about him.

3

A Boy in Vienna

The *Glockengasse* section into which Jacob and Amalia Freud moved with their two children when first they came to Vienna was neither picturesque nor charming. The most that could be said for it was that it was not quite a slum. Jacob found it difficult to establish himelf in business, and Sigmund, as any child of four would, found the change from Freiberg's spaciousness to the stuffy, crowded apartment bewildering.

As a man, he could recall no more than two episodes from these earliest years in Vienna. When he was five his father, in jest, gave him and his sister Anna a book with coloured plates describing a journey through Persia, and bade them tear it up if it so pleased them. The two children blissfully attacked their job of destruction. The only other memory he retained from this period is one which, curiously enough, also revolves around the theme of destruction. As a boy of six, one of the first lessons his mother taught him was that human beings are made of dust, and must therefore return to dust. The boy distrusted this information. He asked for proof. Then his mother rubbed the palms of her hands together with the same gesture she used in making dumplings, and showed the child the dusty flakes of skin which had thus been rubbed off. Sigmund was astonished, but convinced.

At first the small apartment on the *Glockengasse* had

seemed adequate for the family's needs. But as the years passed, the family grew rapidly. After fourteen years of marriage, Jacob and Amalia had produced seven children, two sons and five daughters. Established finally in a six-room apartment in the Leopoldstadt, another dreary Jewish quarter one step removed from a slum, the father, mother and six children distributed themselves among the three bedrooms. To Sigmund, the only member of the family who rated such privacy, a "cabinet" was allotted—a tiny, airless hall bedroom, to be sure, but a room separate from the rest of the family. While the occupants of the other bedrooms used candles to light their way, Sigmund's cabinet boasted the family's only oil lamp. In this room the boy lived and worked until he became an internee at the General City Hospital.

These privileges were granted the boy by his indulgent mother as naturally and inevitably as if they had been part of his birthright. Sigmund was, of course, a diligent and apt student—he was instructed solely by his self-taught father before he entered the gymnasium—and so needed all the privacy and light he could get. But his mother's devotion was so complete that she could not bring herself to deny him anything, even when his wishes and needs came into conflict with those of the rest of the family. She was, for example, very musical, a talent which had skipped Sigmund, but been passed on to his sister, Anna. When Anna's practising penetrated the quiet of Sigmund's hall bedroom and disturbed him at his studies, he told his mother that either the piano must go or he would. "The piano disappeared," his sister Anna recalled many years later, "and with it, all opportunities for his sisters to become musicians. . . ." This wish for peace and quiet while he was working dominated his whole life, though he was not spoiled or demanding in other respects, being content with the simplest of food, clothing and entertainment. During his teens, the boy rarely joined the family at meals, but took them alone in his room where he pored endlessly over his books.

The friends he began to make when he entered the gymnasium were less boys to play with than boys with whom to study and exchange ideas. These young pedants would disappear into Sigmund's room with scarcely a glance for the rest of the family, there to read and discuss issues, and perhaps to mount the plants and flower specimens which Sigmund had brought back from his frequent walks through the forest and woods near Vienna. Very early in his life in Vienna, Sigmund had discovered its woods. These he roamed with as much enthusiasm and wonder as he had in the beautiful forest of Freiberg.

At the same time that the boy drew delight from the study of the pastoral Viennese countryside, he was being made forcibly aware of the less amiable, fiercer aspects of the society he had been born into. In 1866, when Sigmund was ten, Austria went to war with Prussia. At the North Station in Vienna, Sigmund saw the Austrian wounded arriving home, bloody, groaning, white and staring with shock. This was a sight he never forgot. Four years later, during the Franco-Prussian War, the plants, dried flowers and books were pushed aside on his writing desk to make room for a map of the war area, upon which he followed the progress of the campaign with small flags. At the same time the war engrossed him he became interested in the concept of political liberty as it was represented in the United States of America. In 1873, at the American Pavilion of the World's Fair in Vienna, he had obtained some copies of the American Constitution and the Gettysburg Address. His own native land afforded so few political liberties and free ideas that these documents came to him as a revelation, and he not only learned them by heart, but recited and explained them to his young sisters. Introduced to American ideas, he grew curious about American life, and he became a devoted admirer of Mark Twain, whose works he read as they appeared.

By the time his only brother was born, Sigmund was a staunch believer in right through might. A family council, one of many which the democratic Jacob Freud held with his children to discuss all sorts of matters, was called in order to choose a name for the new child. Sigmund's suggestion won. The boy, he said, should be called Alexander because of that great general's prowess and generosity.

And in support of his nomination, he recited the whole story of the Macedonian's triumph.

Although Sigmund had chosen Alexander the Great as the patron saint of his brother, his own personal hero throughout the years of his adolescence was not Alexander but another general—Hannibal, the great Carthaginian leader who sprang from a Semitic background, and who swore undying hatred of Rome and almost succeeded in destroying it. Many years later Freud attempted to trace the origins of his boyhood hero-worship for Hannibal. He said: "Hannibal . . . had been my favourite hero during my years at the gymnasium; like so many boys of my age, I bestowed my sympathies in the Punic war not on the Romans but on the Carthaginians. Moreover, when I finally came to realize the consequences of belonging to an alien race, and was forced by the anti-Semitic feeling among my classmates to take a definite stand, the figure of the Semitic commander assumed still greater proportions in my imagination. Hannibal and Rome symbolized, in my youthful eyes, the struggle between the tenacity of the Jews and the organization of the Catholic Church. . . . I think I can trace my enthusiasm for the Carthaginian general still further back into my childhood, so that it is probably only an instance of an already established emotional relation being transferred to a new vehicle. One of the first books which fell into my childish hands after I learned to read was Thiers' *Consulate and Empire.* I remember that I pasted on the flat backs of my wooden soldiers little labels bearing the names of the Imperial marshals, and that at that time Masséna (as a Jew, Menasse*) was already my avowed favourite. This preference is doubtless also to be explained by the fact of my having been born, a hundred years later, on the same date. Napoleon himself is associated with Hannibal through the crossing of the Alps. And perhaps the development of this martial ideal may be traced yet farther back, to the first three years of my childhood, to wishes which my alternately friendly and

* The Jewish descent of Masséna is somewhat doubtful, a circumstance, however, which was unknown to the child.

hostile relations with a boy a year older than myself must have evoked in the weaker of the two playmates."[9]

Thus, the child whose aggression and subsequent guilt had been awakened by his earliest playmate, had become the adolescent boy who dreamed of the fighter as the most powerful leader in the war against injustice and oppression. To fight off the yoke of domination by force—this was the Jewish boy's reaction to the phenomenon of anti-Semitism. His classmates, who did not hesitate to persecute him for his Jewishness, were nevertheless fully aware of the uses to which his belligerence could be put. With schoolboy inconsistency, they were not averse to using their butt as their leader. Once, for example, when Sigmund's class decided to revolt in a body against an ignorant and unpopular teacher, he was chosen by popular acclaim to act as spokesman for the group.

But about this time an incident took place which was to stop the fighter in his tracks—or at least to cast a wormy doubt on the proposition that might made right. As the boy who was inspired by Hannibal's deeds recalled in later life: "I might have been ten or twelve years old when my father began to take me with him on his walks, and in his conversation to reveal his views on the things of this world. Thus it was that he once told me the following incident, in order to show me that I had been born into happier times than he: 'When I was a young man, I was walking one Saturday along the street in the village where you were born. I was well-dressed, with a new fur cap on my head. Up comes a Christian, who knocks my cap into the mud, and shouts, "Jew, get off the pavement." '

" 'And what did you do?' (asked the young Hannibal).

" 'I went into the street and picked up the cap,' he calmly replied.

"That," the grown Sigmund Freud recalled, with the emotional detachment that was to characterize his whole later life, "did not seem heroic on the part of the big, strong man who was leading me, a little fellow, by the hand. I contrasted this situation, which did not please me, with another, more in harmony with my sentiments—the scene in which Hannibal's father, Hamilcar Barca, made his son swear before the household altar to take vengeance on the Romans."[10]

What Freud might better have said from the vantage-point of his maturity was that ever since then the worm had entered the apple of Hannibal's glory. For, shocked and disappointed as the boy was by his father's revelation that he had met insult with expediency rather than heroism, he could not fail—rebel as he might against Jacob's wisdom and authority—to be shaken in his beliefs by his father's choice of a path of opposition to the agents of oppression and humiliation. Nor did he fail to resent the fact that his father's birth, and consequently his own, laid him open to such attacks. He insisted that the resplendent image of Hannibal remained undimmed for him. But he was, after all, rooted in the ways of his father, and soon other, less martial supermen began to people his day-dreams. He would be, he dreamed, recalling the prophecy of the Prater restaurant's poet, a minister, a statesman. He would study law and jurisprudence as his close friend at the gymnasium, a boy sowewhat older than himself, was planning to do. He would thus reorder the world—and incidentally undo the damage done to his people—by way of the law, not of the sword.

Not only did this incident shake his conviction in the virtue of meeting fire with fire, but it further shook his faith and admiration for his father. For a sensitive boy who gave all his adolescent fervour to the worship of the strong and the brave, this departure of his father from the halls of the heroes was a leave-taking which never lost its poignancy. Sigmund had been enjoined to honour his father, but Jacob Freud, it was evident to his son, was no Hamilcar Barca. How could he continue in imagination to dream himself a Hannibal if he had sprung from so meek and dispirited a forbear?

Other memories antecedent to this one crowded the mind of Sigmund Freud when he set down to dig for the roots of the disenchantment he felt for his father, but would never wholly admit.

"When I was seven or eight years of age," he wrote in *The Interpretation of Dreams,* "another domestic incident occurred which I remember very well. One evening, before going to bed, I had disregarded the dictates of discretion and had satisfied my needs in my parents' bedroom, and in their presence. Reprimanding me for this delinquency, my father remarked: 'That boy will never amount to anything.' This must have been a terrible affront to my ambitions, for allusions to this scene recur again and again in my dreams, and are constantly coupled with enumerations of my accomplishments and successes, as though I wanted to say: 'You see, I have amounted to something after all'. . . . The whole rebellious content of the dream, which commits *lèse-majesté* and scorns authority, may be traced to a revolt against my father. The sovereign is called the father of his country, and the father is the first and oldest, and for the child the only authority, from whose absolutism the other social authorities have evolved in the course of the history of human civilization."[11]

So the boy, whose instinctive reaction to aggression had been to hit back, took the same revenge when aggression of a different sort was directed against him; this time not physical but emotional. It is true, as Freud implies, that this single evidence of paternal rejection was sufficient to haunt him all his life. It is true, as he further implies, that his single-minded pursuit of greatness and achievement all through his life—"one of the immortal infantile wishes . . . the wish to become great," he was to call it in later life—was an effort to vindicate himself in the eyes of his father. "See what I can do, father," his unresting pen wrote between the lines of volume after volume of brilliant investigation into the origins of human behaviour, "your prediction has not come true. Look at the contributions I am making." And, in a sense, all this achievement constituted a hitting back—represented a revenge on the man who was never able to earn enough money to support his family in comfort. But in a profounder sense, the boy—and indeed the man—never really revolted from his father's authority at all, for if he had really not cared for his father's good opinion, he would never have been driven by the necessity to vindicate himself in his eyes. In the same way that the needle of a compass can point a way and act as a guide, and yet remain fixed within the limits of its magnetic orbit, so Sigmund Freud was free to "revolt," to point a way by his achievement, and yet to remain inextricably caught within the limits of his own magnetic field of conflict.

Involved as the basic emotional situation may have been, there was still another aspect of his tie to his father which complicated it further. That facet was the nagging, harrowing sense of guilt which Freud himself was to recognize in other people as the corollary of an unresolved Œdipus complex. What Sigmund Freud was to uncover in his untiring delving into the soul of mankind, and what has today become widely accepted as a primary psychological common denominator, is the fact that the child not only loves its parents but inevitably feels a sexual craving for its parent of the opposite sex.

Freud recognized this in himself. (Indeed, when he found it necessary to disclose the workings of his own unconscious mind in order to describe the purposeful mechanism of dreams, he said somewhat ruefully, "One has to reveal oneself as the sole villain among all the noble souls with whom one shares the breath of life.") He never forgot and explicitly stated that as a child of two he had been impelled by sexual curiosity to penetrate into his parents' bedroom. Later, at seven, to his father's disgust, he had expressed his jealousy by urinating there in his parents' bedroom, in their secret, sexual sanctuary. By urinating there the child was accomplishing more than one purpose: he was, to be sure, expressing his resentment of the sanctuary by "dirtying" and defiling it; but he was also showing his father that his own male organ was an instrument of power; finally, he was reminding his mother of the same incontrovertible fact.

He recalled, furthermore, when he came to discuss the subject of anxiety dreams, that he himself had not had one for "decades." The only one, indeed, which he could recall dated from his "seventh or eighth year," he said. It was, in other words, a dream related in time, not to say content, to the affair of the bedroom. He dreamed then that his "beloved mother, with a peculiarly calm, sleeping countenance [was] carried into the room and laid on the bed by two or three persons with birds' beaks," and, he adds, "I awoke crying and screaming, and disturbed my parents' sleep." In the course of interpreting his dream nearly forty years later, Freud's associations led him to the recollection that the vulgar expression for sexual intercourse in German is *voegeln*—the German for bird is *vogel*—and that his anxiety "could be traced back, through the repression, to a dark, plainly sexual craving, which had found appropriate expression in the visual content of the dream."[12]

Through another one of his own dreams, in which a former patient of his figured, he recalled that this patient's sexual hostility towards his father in childhood had been at the root of his neurosis. In the dream Freud had identified himself with this patient, and he wrote that the reason for the identification was that "I wanted to make an analogous confession to myself."

So Freud as a man revealed as a truth for himself what he postulated as a truth for all of mankind: the fact that the son is his father's rival for the affections of his mother. But for the child and the boy there was no conscious recognition of this familial rivalry. There were only the equally strong, conflicting instinctual drives; the necessity to love and emulate his father as the source from whom all power flowed, and the necessity to hate and oppose him as the dangerous rival who threatened his own potential manhood.

Inherent in this conflict of Freud's was the inability to take and stand by either position wholeheartedly. Thus it took on the emotional colour of guilt. If the child's instinct told him to hate, then his conscience, his upbringing and his environment preached the moral obligation of love, and if he did ban the repugnant idea of hate from his conscious mind in order to cling to love and obedience as the only proper attitudes, then the choked voice of his instincts nagged him pitilessly.

Critics of Freud and his work have tried to prove that his way of life and all that he accomplished was simply an expression of the conflict between himself and his father. These men would have it that Freud was every bit as ghost-ridden as Hamlet, and that the clank of the ghostly chains binding the son to the father echoed endlessly down the long years of the son's life. Like all attempts to explain a man in terms of one truth basic to his life, this attempt to explain Freud is naïve and inadequate.

The unresolved conflict between Freud and his father is, of course, germane to an understanding of the man and his discoveries. But it is only one—albeit a large one—of the pieces of emotional mosaic that go to make up the picture of the whole man. To attempt to fit all the complex manifestations of Sigmund Freud's mind and spirit into the confines of the Œdipus formula is impossible. No amount of prying into psychological first causes, nor sorting of the basic character components of such a man as Freud, can explain the simple and incontrovertible fact of his genius. The path that genius took can be explained, or at least examined; but to try—as Freud did—to reduce all the mysterious facets of the human personality and character to a deterministic, mechanistic blueprint, is a fruitless endeavour. This is the pre-ordained defeat of the mechanistic psychologist. This is the Freudian *manqué*.

4

The Choice of a Path

At the Sperl Gymnasium, Sigmund Freud sat as "primus" on the first bench for eight years. His memory was prodigious. It was easy for him to repeat verbatim the page of a book he had read, and in his 'teens to write down word for word practically the entire content of scientific lectures once he had heard them. His passion for books, by the time he was graduated from the gymnasium, had evolved from delight in destroying them to delight in collecting them. This bibliophilia, he once said, was the earliest passion of his life. It led him at seventeen to run up a debt at a bookshop which he had no means to settle, and for which his father, hard pressed for money, could find no sympathy.

The boy, ignoring the meagre, uncomfortable conditions of his family's life, was lost in the world of knowledge books afforded him. He read everything that came his way, from Goethe and Shakespeare down to the popular novelists of his day. It was inevitable, then, since German was his native tongue, that he should come subtly to be influenced, alien Jew that he was, by German culture. He was, he recalled, "a green youth full of materialistic doctrines." Nevertheless, he was far more seriously affected by the philosophic temper of his time than he cared to admit. Kant, Fichte, Hegel, Schopenhauer, Nietzsche—all had been impressed by the isolation of the ego and its separation from God. God Himself had been reduced by one German philosopher to the state of a "gaseous vertebrate." The spiritual unity of Catholic Europe had been broken by the ferment and liberation of the mechanical revolution which had set men free only to shake their traditional beliefs, and thus to isolate them. This feeling of isolation was reflected in the philosophers' preoccupation, since Kant, with discovering the true nature of the individual.

But philosophy, along with other "unscientific" expressions of the spirit in this mechanistic age, had fallen into disrepute. Although the boy had a markedly philosophical turn of mind, he carefully curbed his inclination to speculate and generalize. Although his powers of observation and expression were great and he wished secretly to be a kind of Goethe, a great literary artist, he soon suppressed an ambition so unrelated to the scientific mechanistic temper of his time. And yet, no one career attracted him exclusively, for his insatiable desire was the desire for knowledge.

He had decided, however, by the time he was graduated *summa cum laude* from the gymnasium, to become a medical student. This decision he reached not because he felt, then or later, any particular enthusiasm for the career of a physician, but because entering the medical school provided the only practical way of combining the study of natural science with the prospect of making money. For it was natural science, as everyone in Freud's day knew, that would provide the most complete answers and the most valuable discoveries about life.

Darwin's theories had just burst upon a shocked and incredulous world and the seventeen-year-old boy was much interested in them, for, he thought, "they held out hopes of an extraordinary advance in our understanding of the world." But the event that clinched his decision to enter medical school was his hearing, shortly before his graduation in the summer of 1873, Goethe's essay on Nature read aloud at a popular lecture by Professor Carl Bruhl. Professor Bruhl was a man with a thrilling voice and the power to communicate his literary excitement. As he read, passages from the Essay began to engrave themselves on the boy's photographic mind:

"Nature! We are surrounded by her, embraced by her—impossible to release ourselves from her and impossible to enter more deeply into her. . . .

"She creates ever new forms; what exists has never existed before; what has existed returns not again—everything is new and yet always old. . . .

"She dwells in none but children; and the mother, where is she? She is the sole artist. . . .

"There is an eternal life, a coming into being and a movement in her; and yet she goes not forward. She is always changing and there is never a moment when she is at rest. Of staying she has no notion and upon inaction she has laid her curse. . . .

"All mankind is in her and she in all. . . .

"Her children are innumerable. To no one is she niggardly, but she has favourites upon whom she lavishes much and to whom she shows great devotion. . . .

"One obeys her laws even if one resists them; one works with her even if one wants to work against her. . . .

"Her crown is love. Only through it does one draw near her. She creates abysses between all beings and everything will swallow itself up. . . . With a draft or two from love's beaker she compensates for a life of toil and trouble. . . .

"She is everything. . . . She is harsh and gentle, lovely and fearful, weak and all-powerful. All is forever present in her. . . .

"She has set me within. She will also lead me without. I commit myself to her."

So a pantheistic pæan to the glories of nature, a poem, not a treatise, confirmed this child of his century in his choice of a career. Since Goethe could be enlisted on the side of scientific inquiry, since he could inspire the boy with echoes of sentiments he recognized as his own, the path was clear. For in Goethe, who synthesized the spirit of German nineteenth-century culture, Freud recognized a kindred spirit. The kinship was based in the boy's mind not only on Goethe's feeling for nature, but on certain similarities between his life and personality and Goethe's. First, there had been the luxuriant growth of black hair at birth for both, the mystic, vital sign of distinction. Then Goethe, too, had been the child of a young, eighteen-year-old, vivacious mother and an older, rather stern and pedantic father. And Goethe, while he had distilled the experiences of his life into some of the greatest lyrical poetry of world literature, had come to believe that it was his contribution to natural science, not literature, that was his crowning achievement. Goethe thus, as the young Freud already sensed he was destined to be, was torn all his life by the necessity to choose between two avenues of expressing his genius for life—the artistic and the scientific.

This polarity of two opposing expressions of the whole of one great truth is the most striking characteristic of the essay which set Freud's feet on the path of medicine. On the one hand, said Goethe, nature is always new; on the other, infinitely old. On the one hand she is "entire"; on the other, "forever incomplete." We cannot hope to know her in her entirety, therefore we must "commit" ourselves to her. This committal implied the same kind of faith in nature as religion presupposes for God.

By the time young Freud heard Goethe's essay read aloud, he had been made to feel that the God of his father was a dubious good. In his walks in the beautiful forest of Freiberg, and later in the *Wienerwald* and the forests of the Salzkammergut, he had found and felt the same divinity Goethe was eulogizing. He was, for all his determined allegiance to the scientific spirit of his era, a boy who needed faith as much as he did bread. He might fight the need, as he did, but he found the godhead Goethe offered in lieu of the Jewish God an infinitely alluring one. The mellifluous voice of the popular Professor Bruhl evoked and focused all the consciously rejected, unconscious religious yearnings of the boy's spirit.

This spirit was pierced, as it had been and continued to be, by a burning shaft of curiosity. "In the years of my youth," Freud once said retrospectively, "the urgent necessity to understand something of the riddles of this world, and perhaps to contribute something myself to their solution, was overpowering." For the true Germanic child of the last half of the nineteenth century, there was only one way to understand nature and unravel its riddles. This was the age of Darwin in genetics, Mendel in heredity, Gustav Theodor Fechner in the laws of the conservation of energy. It was the age of Lord Lister and the beginnings of bacteriology; of the microscope, the test tube and the galvanometer. Those things which could not be observed, measured, weighed and tested in this new age of the ascendancy of natural science were not worth considering at all.

The social sciences like anthropology and sociology did not exist as we know them today. Experimental psychology was in its infancy. It was an age which emphasized facts, disapproved of speculation. Psychiatry, the study of nervous disorders, was limited to description and classification. Psychotic phenomena were regarded as meaningless deviations from the norm, and there was no connection between the psychology of the normal and psychiatry.

Young Freud, who was moved by the spirit of the age, but moved more compellingly, if not so obviously, by an age-old spirit, chose to investigate the mysteries of nature via the path of science. Even then, however, the boy was clear in his mind. It was human nature, not physical objects, that he wanted to study.

His father, who because of his poverty might have been expected to urge the boy towards a more quickly lucrative profession, offered no objection to his son's choice. Indeed, he had always made it clear, despite the boy's conviction of coercion, that Sigmund must follow his own inclinations. So, in the autumn of 1873, Sigmund Freud entered the University of Vienna.

His first days at the University, with Goethe's fine words ringing in his ears, were ones of bitter disappointment. The anti-Semitism he had encountered in high school pursued him into the halls of the University. He found that he was expected to feel himself inferior and an alien because he was a Jew. He refused, despite the efforts of his classmates, to betray any feeling of inferiority. He protested bravely that he had never been able to see why he should feel ashamed of his descent, or, as people were beginning to say, of his race. He showed no outward regret—whatever his inner feelings may have been—and calmly, quietly, he put up with his non-acceptance into the fellowship of students. His work, he decided, was more important than the prejudices of his classmates.

Determined as he was to ignore his enforced isolation, he was not unaffected by it. "At an early age," he said of these days, "I was made familiar with the fate of being in the opposition and of being put under the ban of the 'compact majority.' The foundations were thus laid for a certain degree of independence of judgment." The foundations he thus dates had, of course, been laid long before then. What was newly laid was a supporting stone in his will towards self-sufficiency—a reinforced determination to stand alone if he could not stand together. He would make his Jewishness, the cause of his vulnerability and isolation, into a strength. He would show his tormentors what a Jew could do. Although this necessity to vindicate himself in the eyes of society, which echoed his necessity to vindicate himself in the eyes of his father, was to become one of his greatest sources of strength, it contained at the same time the seeds of his weakness: his resentment, secret and unacknowledged, at being a Jew at all, at being forced to feel inferior when he was convinced of his own superior endowments.

For three years Freud floundered at the University, going from department to department in the natural sciences, seeking the one branch which would best help him to find the answers to the questions which gave him no rest. At chemistry he worked diligently but unfruitfully, and he was humiliated by his failure to accomplish anything in what he called "that exacting science." Zoology proved equally unrewarding.

These years of introduction to the scientific world were broken up by a nostalgic experience—his first journey beyond the borders of Austria and his only voluntary trip to England. Freud was nineteen when, as a reward from his father for his splendid school record, he went to Manchester to visit his two half-brothers. This was for him the renewal of the old ties with Emmanuel and John—a renewal made happier by the fact that they were now all men together. Emmanuel was surprised and pleased with Sigmund and wrote to Jacob in Vienna: "You have given me great pleasure in sending us Sigmund. He is a splendid spectacle of a fine human being, and if I had the pen of a Dickens, I could well make a hero of him." Sigmund, in his turn, got from long conversations with Emmanuel a new, less bitter perspective on his father. He learned something of the difficulties of his father's young life. But the best of his new experiences was the fact that for the first time he was living in an atmosphere different from what he had known. For a short time, he was not a Jew in a German-speaking land, and the experience was for him both strange and enjoyable.

Home again in 1876 and back at the University, he at last hit upon a branch of science and a teacher which seemed to provide an answer to what he had been seeking. He found rest and satisfaction in Ernst Bruecke's physiological laboratory, and he found, also, men to whom he could look up: the eminent Bruecke himself and his assistants, Sigmund Exner and Ernst von Fleischl-Marxow. With the brilliant Fleischl, Freud became friendly. He grew so enthusiastic about his work and teachers in the laboratory that he forgot temporarily such matters as degrees and graduation, and remained with Bruecke for six years, until 1882.

The influence of the venerable Ernst Bruecke, "the Helmholtzian ambassador to the Far East"—that is, to Vienna—was, as a scientist and as a man, significant to the development of the budding scientist. The physiology which Bruecke taught stemmed in a direct line from the physicist Robert Mayer's great discoveries about the conservation of energy.* Within twenty-five years of the date of Mayer's discovery, the Helmholtz school which applied these discoveries to the physiology of the nervous system had achieved virtual domination over the thinking and

* There was another physicist whose work influenced Freud strongly—Gustav Theodor Fechner, whose psychophysical law of the conservation of energy Freud was later to apply to psychology.

teaching of the German physiologists and medical teachers, and in so doing had not only contributed further important solutions to age-old scientific puzzles, but had provided great impetus to science everywhere.

In the 1860s, students in German universities were as interested in and stimulated by the "new" Helmholtzian theories as students today are by the implications of nuclear fission. When Freud entered medical school in 1873, the Helmholtz furor had passed its peak. But the study of physiology was still pervaded by it, and Bruecke's Physiological Institute was still active, famous and glamorous.

Bruecke was a man whose entire life was filled by his science. Among the great investigators of his time whose forte was the painstaking observation and description of natural phenomena, Bruecke's genius, mechanical as it might seem from a modern standpoint, was compelling. "Those who had worked under Bruecke," Fritz Wittels, a disciple of Freud's, once wrote, "might subsequently become interested in fields remote from physiology, but they could never forget what they had learned about the scientific method." Bruecke's eyes were cold, blue, piercing and, in Freud's dreams where they later turned up, "formidable." It is likely that the eyes which lived on in Freud's dream life twenty-five years later symbolized to him the scientific caution and exactitude whose necessity had been impressed upon him so forcibly by Bruecke.

Bruecke's assistant, Ernst von Fleischl-Marxow, the man with whom the young Freud found it a privilege to be friendly, was an even more fanatical scientist than his master. His life at the time Freud studied under him had already become a tormenting progress of pain and inevitably approaching death. Yet he continued to pursue his work with vigour, brilliance and constancy. This path of single-minded scientific dedication must have strongly impressed the young Freud, for it was the path he himself was to follow when pain and imminent death confronted him.

Bruecke and Fleischl were, Freud later said, the first teachers in his field whom he "could respect and take as . . . models." In other words, these were the men fanatically devoted to scientific investigation, who best fitted in with Freud's already well-formed ideas of selfless dedication to a cause. They were the men he could emulate. That Freud at twenty, and even at twenty-five, dispossessed of the ideal image of his father, needed idols to reverence and pattern himself after, is not surprising. Bruecke and Fleischl were replacements for Masséna, Hannibal and the great men of jurisprudence who had occupied the altars of his boyhood. Boy or man, however, heroes and hero-worship remained essential to Freud.

With his hopes fixed longingly but blindly on research as a career, Freud spent six of the happiest years of his youth immersed in study in Bruecke's laboratory. He worked on the problems which Bruecke had set him—first a problem in the histology of the nervous system which he not only succeeded in solving to Bruecke's satisfaction, but carried further on his own account; and then an investigation of the spinal cord of one of the lowest forms of fish, *Ammacoetes Petroyyxon*. Preoccupied with the nervous system of this fish, he paid little attention to the rest of his medical curriculum. Indeed, other branches of medicine proper, with the exception of psychiatry, held little interest for him. Thus it was not until 1881—eight years where it normally required five to complete the course—that he took his belated degree as a Doctor of Medicine.

There had been another, and a good, reason for his dilatory progress towards his degree. Both he and his fellow students had assumed, so marked was Bruecke's interest in him, that he was slated to fill the next post of assistant that fell vacant in the laboratory. He had, as a matter of fact, every right to count on becoming Bruecke's assistant. He had worked with diligence and originality on the problems Bruecke had assigned him. He had met favour and promise in the master's stern blue eye. He had worked neglecting his other studies, on the implicit assumption that he had found his niche and would spend the rest of his life pursuing Bruecke's path of abstract, theoretical research.

The shock must have been great when early in 1882 Bruecke advised him to abandon the laboratory and the life it meant. There would be no assistant's post for him. Bruecke told him, and he had best forget his career in theoretical research altogether, lest he remain poor all his life. With the gate to a career to which the young man had already devoted six years' work so firmly slammed in his face, Freud had no choice but to agree.

The necessity of earning money, which he had disregarded in fine scholarly fashion throughout his university career, was now in any case a matter of concern. In all these years of single-minded study he had been financed by his father, who could ill afford the luxury of a son who could not support himself. His father might be willing to subsidize him indefinitely, but upon graduation Freud had become engaged to marry Martha Bernays, a girl whose family came from Hamburg and whose brother Ely was about to marry Sigmund's sister, Anna. In order to marry, Freud needed to pick up the threads of the general medical career he had dropped in his absorption with the physiological laboratory.

So he followed Bruecke's advice, left the laboratory and entered Vienna's principal hospital, the *Allgemeine Krankenhaus*, as an "aspirant" or internee. Soon afterwards he became a junior resident physician working in various departments of the hospital. There, as at the University, he found a man and a branch of science which claimed his devotion and homage. The man was the renowned psychiatrist, Dr. Theodor Meynert, with whose work and personality Freud had been impressed while still a student. The work was cerebral anatomy, and in Meynert's Institute of Cerebral Anatomy Freud worked with as much concentration for six months as he had for six years in physiology under Bruecke.

In a way, however, he remained faithful to the line of work he had originally undertaken. His project under Bruecke had been the study of the spinal cord of one of the lowest of the fishes. Under Meynert, Freud proceeded to the study of the central nervous system of the human. In contrast to the diffuse character of his studies during his undergraduate days, he developed an inclination to concentrate his work exclusively on a single subject or problem—at first, in this case, the medulla oblongata. This inclination to concentrate was to persist with such intensity that it led eventually to the charge of Freud's one-sidedness.

The medulla oblongata was interesting, but brain anatomy could be considered no more practical than physiology, and with the idea of earning enough income to permit his marriage, Freud began to study nervous diseases. At that time there were few specialists in that branch of medicine in Vienna. The study of nervous diseases was distributed over a number of different departments in the hospital. Even Professor Nothnagel, who had received his appointment in psychiatry a short time before Freud started his studies, on account of his book on cerebral localization, did not find it necessary to single out neuropathology from other subdivisions of medicine. In short, Freud was convinced that he must be his own teacher if he wanted to specialize as a practitioner in nervous diseases. In this psychiatric desert, there shone for Freud the distant glittering name of Charcot, which stood for whatever progress and experimentation was taking place in the field. He soon decided first to obtain an appointment as Lecturer in Nervous Diseases in Vienna, and then to save enough money to go to Paris to continue his studies under Charcot.

Meynert, to be sure, had previously made Freud an offer: he had suggested that Freud devote himself exclusively to the study of the anatomy of the brain, and in return he would hand over to him the lecturing work in anatomy which he was beginning to feel too old to handle. This offer, which would have meant so much to Freud a few years previously, he declined—"in alarm," he said later, "at the magnitude of the task. It is possible too that I had guessed already that this great man was by no means kindly disposed towards me." This "guess" was later borne out.*

* Meynert the friend and patron became his enemy once Freud began to experiment with hypnosis and the early stages of psychoanalysis. Like the return of a major theme in a symphony comes the sound of Freud's words of self-analysis: "An intimate friend and a

During the years Freud was an internee at the *Allgemeine Krankenhaus* he published a number of papers on organic diseases of the nervous system. His skill as a clinician and diagnostician was developing. He was able, for example, to localize the site of a lesion in the medulla oblongata so accurately that the pathological anatomist found nothing to correct. He was the first physician in Vienna to send a case for autopsy with a diagnosis of polyneuritis acuta. The fame of his diagnoses soon brought him an influx of American doctors to whom Freud lectured on the cases in his department in a kind of pidgin English.

But for all his clinical ability, he understood, so far, nothing about the neuroses. Once he introduced to his audience a neurotic suffering from a persistent headache as a case of chronic localized meningitis. His students laughed at him, and, says Freud, "my premature activities as a teacher came to an end." The young doctor, however, made this mistake at a time when older and more distinguished physicians than he were habitually diagnosing neurotic conditions as cerebral tumour.

Despite this pedagogical humiliation, Freud was appointed Lecturer on Neuropathology at the hospital in the spring of 1885—largely because of the excellence of his biological and clinical publications. A few months later, on the strength of a glowing recommendation from Bruecke, he was awarded a travelling fellowship whose value was sufficient to take him to Charcot and Paris. The glimmering in the distance had become a reality. Freud was to find in Paris, the second foreign city he had ever visited, the clue which would lead him to his own original contribution to psychiatry.

---

hated enemy have always been indispensable to my emotional life; I have always been able to create them anew, and not infrequently my childish ideal has been so closely approached that friend and enemy have coincided in the same person."

5

Paris in the Spring

The slight, slender, twenty-nine-year-old Freud, black of hair and eye, felt lost and anonymous in the crowd of students who had flocked to Paris from all over Europe. He began his studies immediately at the Salpêtrière, the Parisian insane asylum which, through the work of Jean Marie Charcot, had become the Mecca for Europe's most progressive neurologists and psychiatrists.

Charcot's important contribution to medical psychiatry had been his success in making the use of hypnotism respectable in medical practice. Mesmerism, from which hypnotism evolved, had long been regarded as charlatanry in scientific circles, as superstitious as astrology, alchemy and demonology. However, in the middle of the nineteenth century an English physician and a French country doctor, A. A. Liébeault, had begun to use hypnotic sleep successfully as a method of treatment and research. Liébeault's fame spread, and in Paris, in 1878, Charcot established the Salpêtrière school of hypnosis, an institution devoted to investigating, systematizing and classifying all existent knowledge about the phenomenon.

In 1882, three years before Freud's arrival, Charcot had achieved his greatest coup: the French Academy of Sciences, which had condemned all research on animal magnetism not once but three times, accepted with interest his long description of hypnotic phenomena. This nod from the Academy brought to an end once and for all the interminable controversy over magnetism. This constituted a momentous occasion in the history of medical psychiatry, for it put an end to the taboo which had been holding back research in psychiatry and reopened a territory for exploration which had long been closed. Thus hypnotism, rescued from limbo, had become a fully accredited medical tool by the eighteen-eighties, when it was being used both as a method of treatment and as a method of research. It was also itself a subject of research. But all attempts to understand it and all the deeper psychological aspects of suggestibility were not successful with the methods then available. Charcot, who was a thoroughly trained neurologist, and whose studies of hypnotism had started from his work with pathological anatomy, taught primarily in terms of the physical action of the nervous system. The method of investigation he used explored the nature of the changes occurring in the brain and nerves during hypnotic states. He worked painstakingly and accumulated much information, but he reached the conclusion that hypnotic states could be induced only in those people who suffered from hysteria. So he considered the phenomenon of hypnotism a manifestation of abnormality. Under these circumstances the nature of hypnotism remained demonstrable but baffling.

"Hysteria," whose name had derived from the Greek root *hysteron*, meaning uterus, was universally considered to be an organic disorder of the womb. The psychiatrists of the 'eighties worked on the assumption that the organic existence of the disease was not to be questioned, and that the sole job of the rational physician was to study its nature and development. As late as 1882, a reputable French physician removed the ovary of a patient in order to cure hysteria, and at about the same time physicians in Vienna, London and Heidelberg were engaged in the surgical removal and cauterization of the clitoris in similar attempts.

Although Charcot took no particular interest in fully investigating the psychology of hysteria, nevertheless he remained convinced that hysterical symptoms were by-products of an organic, morbid cause combined with hereditary predisposition. Conclusive proof of this organic origin was notably lacking, but the physiological orientation of the day remained the only direction in which the Charcot school allowed itself to look.

Despite the limitations, from a post-Freudian vantage-point, of Charcot's outlook, his demonstrations at the Salpêtrière were both popular and authoritative. His was the first centre of postgraduate psychiatric education, an immensely significant advance since the graduate work of the physician of the time included no psychiatry. And the existence of Charcot's school, under the protective wing of an established hospital and medical school, gave tremendous impetus to the further study of neuroses, a study which had for too long been ignored.

Freud knew no one in Paris. He would take his lonely walks to and from the hospital, back and forth from his solitary lodgings, and "frequently," he said later, "I . . . heard my name suddenly pronounced by an unmistakable dear voice. . . . I then made a note of the exact moment of the hallucination in order to inquire carefully of those at home what had occurred at the time."[13] His scientific preoccupation with the hallucinations produced by homesickness, and his longing for his fiancée, were not enough to occupy his loneliness. He longed on his solitary walks, he says, "for a helper and protector." And he spun daydreams in which he hurled himself at a runaway horse, bringing it to a standstill, and the great personage occupying the carriage stepped out, pressed his hand and said, "You are my saviour—I owe my life to you! What can I do for you?"

The fantasies and the longing for protection were completely at variance with his desire to play the strong man himself. But his first long residence completely away from his family, his utter solitude, reawakened in him a need for warmth and protection. Although a little later he professed, and was able to act out, a deep-rooted scorn at the idea of being someone's protégé, at the moment, fresh from the sterilized arms of Bruecke and Meynert, that was exactly what he wanted to be. He soon set about remedying his solitary situation. He wrote to Charcot and suggested that he, Freud, translate Charcot's new volume of lectures into German. Charcot accepted. One meeting led to another, and soon Freud became a member of Charcot's circle, and a leading participant in all that went on at the clinic.

Freud was much impressed with Charcot. The man's methods provided as memorable and instructive a lesson as working with Bruecke had been. Freud was fascinated not only by hypnotism, but by the dynamics of hysteria, and Charcot's demonstrations of the effect of hypnotic suggestion on hysterical subjects, the ease with which he could produce hysterical symptoms in these people under hypnosis and then remove the symptoms by the same method, interested Freud greatly. He was also struck by the fact that these artifically produced symptoms reproduced down to their smallest details the same features as the genuine attacks which Charcot had not induced. He noted, too, that many of Charcot's hysterical subjects were men, a startling enough circumstance to a member of a scientific generation which believed that hysterical phenomena arose from the disordered womb. And he was interested to learn that hysterical or psychic phenomena could be described, arranged and classified and could conform to the rigid regularities of scientific law in the same way as the anatomical and physiological data he had so diligently studied under Bruecke and Meynert.

It was not only Charcot's procedure which impressed Freud. He was also fascinated by Charcot's personality. One day when Charcot was being heckled by his students, who questioned his ability to prove one of the theories he was expounding, he jumped up and down and cried impatiently, "*Cela n'empêche pas d'exister.*"[7] In other words, the fact that no empirical proof could be offered did not, in Charcot's mind, impair the validity of a theory he *felt* to be true. This remark of Charcot's left what Freud called "an indelible mark" on his mind, and when Freud came in later years to evaluate the position of Charcot in his own scientific life, he said, with admiration: "He was not a thinker, but a man of artistic temperament—to use his own word—a 'seer'. He told us about the way he worked. It was his practice with things that were new to him to look at them again and again, intensifying the impression of them from day to day, until suddenly and spontaneously understanding would come. Before his mental vision, chaos would change into order, and the change would always occur along the same lines. He would grow aware of the existence of new types of disease, characterized by the constant association of symptoms in particular groups. . . . He would say that the greatest delight a man could experience was to see something new—that is to recognize it as new."[14]

Freud himself was to pursue his own investigations in much the same fashion. The words he wrote about Charcot he might well have written about himself. Charcot's example gave Freud the courage to use his own innate gifts as a "seer" without fear of scientific opprobrium. From another of his heroes Freud had assimilated a lesson worth learning.

Freud stayed in Paris from the autumn of 1885 to the spring of 1886. Membership in Charcot's circle, rewarding though it might be, was hardly the society he longed for. Martha Bernays had been waiting for him for four years. Despite the dilatory ardour this long wait implied, it is to be presumed that he was eager to marry, and that his blood stirred at the thought of Martha, distant though she was. Caution, learned at some cost, had dictated the completion of his studies before he settled down with a wife. Now as his time in Paris drew to a close and the chestnut trees began to bud, his restlessness overcame him. The possibility of sexual gratification outside the bounds of matrimony would have been morally repugnant to him.

Instead, he sought the Cathedral. Every free afternoon he had he would go up into the towers of Notre Dame, "and there clamber about between the monsters and gargoyles." What he dreamed of, perched on this pinnacle of the Christian world, he never revealed. Knowledge, heroism, achievement, fame, love? In all likelihood, it was most often love, for in his susceptible condition he was wistfully envious of the tender temper of Paris. He remembered for years how on a spring day on the Boulevard St. Michel he had seen a group of young men and women walking in front of him. Every now and then they would stop walking and start spontaneously to dance without any apparent cause or motive, but just because they were young and in Paris and it was springtime.

With all his longing thoughts of Martha, he was a little aghast at the idea of assuming the responsibility of a wife and family. All of his life so far had been spent in the cloistered pursuit of study. He had never earned enough by the age of thirty to support himself, let alone a family. Would he be able, he wondered, to make enough money as a specialist in nervous diseases? And if he did, if he was to become just another ordinary practitioner, which he had never wanted to be, what of his ambitions to create, to contribute something to the understanding of the world?

He was beginning to feel that a wife would deflect him from his purpose. Somehow, although he was prepared to admit his unreasonableness, he felt that his fiancée had already kept him from becoming famous. The year before he came to Paris, a side interest had led him to the study of what was then a little known alkaloid compound—cocaine. In the midst of this work an opportunity had arisen for him to visit Martha, whom he had not seen for two years. He wound up his investigation of cocaine in haste, and contented himself in his monograph on the subject with the prophecy that future uses would undoubtedly be found for it. Before he left he told his friend Koenigstein, the ophthalmologist, and Carl Koller about the compound, and suggested to them that its anæsthetizing properties might conceivably be useful in diseases of the eye. Then he departed for Hamburg and Martha.

Upon his return, he was surprised and dismayed to find that Koller had followed up his suggestion, made the decisive experiments on animals' eyes, and demonstrated the uses of the drug to the Ophthalmological Congress at Heidelberg. Koller was therefore considered to be the discoverer of local anæsthesia by cocaine, which at the time became quite important in minor surgery. Freud, after relating the details of this incident in his *Autobiography*, winds up his account by saying, "But I bore my fiancée no grudge for her interruption of my work."

The fact remains that he *did* bear her a grudge. His loss of the credit for the discovery of cocaine's anæsthetic properties rankled even after he had become known as the discoverer of psychoanalysis. As late as 1906, in his lectures on his new science to his early disciples, he would remind his listeners that he was the rightful discoverer of cocaine. In his dreams, the cocaine episode also figured. Sixteen years after the event, in the course of interpreting one of his dreams, he was reminded of the monograph he had written on cocaine: "I had hinted that the alkaloid might be employed as an anæsthetic," he said, "but I was not thorough enough to pursue the matter further." He then recounted a fantasy he had on the morning of the day after this dream: "I had thought of cocaine in a kind of daydream," he said. "If I were ever afflicted with glaucoma, I would go to Berlin, and there undergo an operation, incognito, in the house of my Berlin friend, at the hands of a surgeon whom he would recommend. The surgeon, who would not know the name of his patient, would boast as usual how easy these operations had become since the introduction of cocaine; and I should not betray the fact that I myself had a share in this discovery. . . . Only after recalling this day-dream do I realize that there is concealed behind it the memory of a definite event. Shortly after Koller's discovery, my father contracted glaucoma; he was operated on by my friend Dr. Koenigstein, the eye specialist. Dr. Koller was in charge of the cocaine anæsthetization, and he made the remark that on this occasion all the three persons who had been responsible for the introduction of cocaine had been brought together."[15]

The fact that Martha had been the unwitting agent of his failure to be credited with the discovery of cocaine continued to affront Freud's ambition and his need for prestige for a long time. He certainly regretted the fact that he had allowed sentiment to interfere with the pursuit of his career, particularly since his career at this juncture was so uncertain. Still not clear in his mind as to the exact nature of the contribution he felt destined to make, he was loath to relinquish whatever minor claim to fame might come his way. It is evident, too, that the cocaine episode assumed the aspect of a major disappointment in Freud's mind partly because it coincided with his father's affliction by glaucoma. Cocaine had been used in his father's operation. Cocaine had therefore been the first tangible means whereby the son had helped his father, and had demonstrated the falseness of the paternal taunt that he would never amount to anything. This, Freud recognized. In discussing another of his dreams in which a man afflicted with glaucoma figured, he said, "By means of the glaucoma I reminded my father of cocaine, which stood him in good stead during his operation, as though I had thereby fulfilled my promise." Since he was not the accredited discoverer of cocaine, he had not proved his worth to his father beyond the shadow of a doubt. He was not able to enter this first of his achievements in the long mental list of successes he felt driven to present to his father. No wonder it seemed to him, despite his impatience to marry, that Martha had, in some subtle sense, wronged him.

Martha, who had waited obediently for more than four years, had not much longer to wait—only a few months while Freud detoured to Berlin on his way home, there to gain more knowledge of the diseases of childhood. Marriage was important and his need clamoured for fulfillment, but his thirst for knowledge seems to have been even more insistent. Before he went to Paris he had been promised a position heading the department of children's nervous diseases at the Kassowitz Institute, a Viennese hospital for children. He felt it was necessary to prepare himself for practice in this field before he was free to settle down to matrimony and the obligations of family life.

At last, in the autumn of 1886, the prolonged courtship came to an end. With Freud established finally but precariously in Vienna as a specialist in nervous diseases, the marriage took place. The young couple seemed to be scornful of superstition, for they set up housekeeping in a place the rest of Vienna shunned like the plague—the *Suehnhaus*, or the House of Atonement, as the Viennese called it. This was an apartment house built on the site of the State Theatre, which had recently burned down with a loss of six hundred lives. The young Freuds, too determinedly rational to be discouraged by the aura of doom which hung over the place, were among the first to rent an apartment there. There their first child, Mathilda, was born in 1887—an event commemorated by the Emperor Franz Josef, who honoured this first born of the *Suehnhaus* with a handsome commemorative vase from the Royal Porcelain Workshops.

Freud's wife, like his mother, came from a family which included scholars and intellectuals famous in Jewish culture. Martha Bernays Freud's grandfather, Isaac Bernays, had been chief rabbi of Hamburg during the great reform movement which swept orthodox Judaism around 1848. This liberal tide he had fought determinedly. Isaac Bernays was mentioned frequently in Heinrich Heine's letters as a "*geistreicher Mann*," an upright man of high intelligence. Another Bernays edited the *Vorwaerts*, a radical German language newspaper published in Paris in the early eighteen-forties, which first printed some of Heine's poems. Heine once ask to be remembered to this Bernays in a letter to Karl Marx, who also contributed to the *Vorwaerts*. Jacob and Michael, Isaac's sons, taught at German universities—Jacob taught Latin and Greek at Heidelberg and Michael became a professor of German at Munich. Jacob, who clung unswervingly to the orthodox faith of his father, never attained a full professorship, for it was virtually impossible for a Jew in a German university to achieve this pedagogic distinction. He did, however, gain scholarly renown. His works are still esteemed and used by classical philologists. Michael Bernays, on the other hand, embraced an opportunism that he felt would advance his career. He renounced his religion, embraced Christianity, and won his full professorship at Munich. Later he rose to a position of unprecedented honour for a man born the son of a Jew.

He became confidant and *Lehr-Konsul,* a kind of official reader, to the mad King Ludwig of Bavaria. Among his other achievements was a weighty but unimpressive book on Goethe.

Jacob, following the ancient Jewish custom, went into full mourning for Michael when he renounced his faith. A third brother, Martha Bernays' father, no intellectual but a merchant, read the apostate out of the family. Many years later, when Michael Bernays came to her city to deliver a lecture, Martha Bernays was forced to sneak secretly out of his father's house to hear him, for even so passive an association with heresy was strictly forbidden to the children of this brother's family.

In this atmosphere of tight orthodoxy, under the wing of a sternly righteous father, Martha Bernays grew up. She was raised in the cool, formal atmosphere of Hamburg. The icy blasts blowing from the North Sea over the port city of Hamburg seemed to have imparted a measure of their frigidity to the character of the city's inhabitants, just as the glistening, lazy Danube seemed to have coloured the character of the people of Vienna.

Not that Martha Bernays was any more an undiluted product of Hamburg than Sigmund Freud was of Vienna. But Martha was sufficiently influenced by her Hamburg upbringing to remain something of an anomaly in the easy, gregarious life of Vienna. The precision of her speech and manner, which suggested the governess—her maiden sister, Minna, who soon became a member of the Freuds' household, had indeed been a governess—clicked in marked contrast to the slurred and colourful Viennese dialect. At the beginning, it occurred neither to her nor to "Tante" Minna to make the slightest concession to the temper and style of life in Vienna. And after fifty years of living in Vienna, both ladies still spoke the brand of "pure" German for which Hamburg is noted, a circumstance which often got them into difficulties, for to the tradespeople of Vienna their speech sounded almost like a foreign language.

The aloofness which marked Martha Freud and her sister, whose rôle in the household became almost as important, was not born of the difference in language alone. In innumerable little mannerisms, habits and orderly traditions, the two Hamburg ladies ran Freud's home so that to one impressionable observer it "gave me an impression of extraterritoriality, like an island that is easily accessible from the mainland, but still an island." Small, lithe and as quickly active as a wren, Martha Freud epitomized the cleaning, brushing, tidying *hausfrau* who neither rests nor wishes to while a cushion still remains to be plumped.

Although six children, three boys and three girls, were born to the Freuds within the first ten years of their marriage, Martha Freud organized the household to revolve around the convenience of *der Papa,* as the children referred to their father. As fixed and immutable as a timetable, each household event was arranged to come off with promptness, accuracy and dispatch. *Mittagessen* was served promptly at one o'clock, and woe to the tardy child who showed such disrespect for the excellent food and for Papa's schedule.

While the household and all who lived in it were rigidly regimented to move only in their prescribed orbits around the sun who was *der Papa,* Frau Freud oiled the incomparably efficient household machinery with the measured, temperate kindliness that was natural to her. Tante Minna, Frau Freud's maiden sister, might be more forthright and more aggressive. She might lend to her few, pungent words a decidedly epigrammatic turn. She might understand more clearly the importance of the work Sigmund Freud was doing, and she might in time come to act as his secretary. Certainly she had more time for, and was fonder of reading and could evaluate what she read with discrimination and wit. But her slimmer, smaller sister, who had neither the time nor the zest for intellectual pursuits, had a kind of deep, albeit restrained and delimited humanity to offer in place of Minna's more clearly defined individuality. Attached as Frau Freud was to her household effects, she never let them take precedence over the welfare of a servant. Servants stayed on and on in the Freud house, and at Christmas Frau Freud's long list included not only all the household servants, but all the relatives of all the people who served the house in any way. Minna's acerb comment on her sister's Christmas solicitude was typical. "We draw the line only at the niece of our milkman," she said.

Sigmund Freud, in short, had married a worthy woman who typified the homely traditional virtues of her people and her society. It could not be said that she was either lusty, passionate or her husband's intellectual equal. On the other hand, she would provide for him—if not with the same degree of overt warmth—the same care and devotion to his physical comfort which his mother had shown him. And with his wife, as with his mother, the first women in his life, he would come first. His needs, his desires, his wishes would remain, as in his mother's house, the pivot around which the rest of the family, including his wife, revolved. Nor, since it is to be assumed that the restraint and detachment of her outward manner did not conceal a violently emotional heart, would she challenge the supremacy of the deep, warm bond that Freud had felt first for his mother. It is in any case likely, given her character and personality, that she was as much a victim of sexual inhibitions and taboos as other women of her Victorian time. If this is not, in outline, the basic psychological foundation for Freud's marriage, it would be strange and difficult indeed to understand the course that marriage took.

6

La Chose Genitale

As a practising physician, Freud at first met nothing but trouble and opposition. As soon as he advised the conservative members of the Vienna Medical Society of his newfangled French notions, he was greeted with scorn. He delivered a report to that Society on what he had seen and learned in Charcot's laboratory, and he touched upon the hysterical men who had been under observation there. Immediately an elderly surgeon interrupted him testily.

"My dear sir," he said, "how can you talk such nonsense? *Hysteron* means the uterus, so how can a man be hysterical?"

When Freud found and demonstrated a hysterical man to the Society he was applauded, but, he says, "no further interest was taken in me." The high dignitaries of Viennese medicine rejected his innovations by ignoring them. He found that, with his theory of hysteria in men and his production of hysterical paralysis by suggestion, he was just as thoroughly shunned by the "compact majority" as he had ever been in his university days.

Soon afterwards, Meynert, his former patron at the Institute of Cerebral Anatomy, who declared that hypnosis was nothing more than a method for the artificial production of imbecility, excluded Freud from his laboratory.*

* For this exclusion Meynert, who had now become Freud's enemy, was repaid. In the course of analysing one of his own dreams in *The*

Thus Freud was left with no place to deliver his lectures, and was forced to withdraw almost entirely from academic life and from attendance at the learned medical societies.

As far as his practice was concerned, his "therapeutic arsenal contained only two weapons," he said, "electrotherapy and hypnotism, for prescribing a visit to a hydropathic establishment after a single consultation was an inadequate source of income." The standard textbook on electrotherapy at the time was Erb's. It was treated as a bible, but Freud found it a "construction of fantasy." "The realization that the work of the greatest name in German neuropathology," he said, "had no more relation to reality than some 'Egyptian' dream book, such as is sold in cheap bookshops, was painful, but it helped to rid me of another shred of the innocent faith in authority from which I was not yet free."[16]

That left hypnotism, which the Viennese brotherhood of psychiatrists branded as not only fraudulent, but dangerous. Hypnotists, despite the growing recognition accorded Charcot, were still regarded beyond the pale and with the coldest scientific contempt. Strengthened in his independence by the fact that he was already beyond the pale in any case, Freud for the first five years of his practice used hypnotic suggestion as his principal instrument. He found, as he says, "there was something positively seductive in working with hypnotism." It gave him for the first time a sense of having overcome his helplessness in the face of phenomena whose meaning eluded him. His capitulation

---

Interpretation of Dreams, he wrote: "The great Meynert, in whose footsteps I followed with such veneration, and whose attitude towards me, after a short period of favouritism, changed into one of undisguised hostility. The dream recalls to me his own statement that in his youth he formed the habit of intoxicating himself with chloroform, with the result that he had to enter a sanatorium; and also my second experience with him shortly before his death. I had a literary controversy with him in reference to masculine hysteria, the existence of which he denied, and when I visited him during his last illness, and asked him how he felt, he described his condition at some length, and concluded with the words: 'You know, I have always been one of the prettiest cases of masculine hysteria.' Thus, to my satisfaction and to my astonishment, he admitted what he so long and so stubbornly denied."

to the sweet seduction of hypnotism meant that he would have to abandon the treatment of people suffering from organic nervous diseases. This he was ready to do, for the prospect of making money in the treatment of such disorders had never been especially promising. With his family increasing rapidly, Freud needed money. Moreover, the number of nervous patients suffering organically was slight compared to the crowds of neurotics whose number seemed to Freud "further multiplied by the manner in which they hurried, with their troubles unsolved, from one doctor to another." What is more, his success with the method was steadily gaining him a reputation which the disapproval of official medical circles could do little to affect. He was pleased and flattered at the reputation of a miracle-worker he was beginning to enjoy.

Neurotics flocked to Freud's office. In treating them he was forced to recognize the drawbacks of hypnotism: he was unable to hypnotize every patient he wished to, and he was unable to put certain patients into as deep a hypnotic state as he wanted. Because of what he felt to be shortcomings in his own technique of hypnosis, he thought he needed further study. At Nancy, in France, a medical school had been established which was using extensively and with considerable therapeutic success, not hypnotism solely, but suggestion with or without hypnotism. In the summer of 1889 Freud set out for Nancy to see for himself what the Doctors Liébeault and Bernheim were doing to expand the frontiers of psychotherapy.

In two rooms in a corner of his garden at Nancy, Liébeault ran a clinic into which the poor people of the neighbourhood crowded, not because they understood the principle that physical disorders could be caused by mental disturbance, but because Liébeault was able to cure them. Liébeault was an unassuming, hard-working country doctor who, settling in Nancy in 1864, had gradually begun to use hypnotic sleep for treatment and research. Beloved and trusted by the poor, who called him *le bon père Liébeault,* he understood how to make the simple people co-operate with him. "If you wish me to treat you with drugs," he would tell them, "I will do so, but you will have to pay me as before. But if you will allow me to hypnotize you, I will do it for nothing." Thus Liébeault in his shrewd and modest way was effecting cures by the use of hypnotism.

Bernheim had visited Liébeault in 1882 to find out how he had cured a stubborn case of sciatica with which Bernheim had grappled six months with no success. Impressed by what he saw of Liébeault's methods, he became his friend and pupil and began to apply Liébeault's principles to his own hospital patients. Like *le bon père*, his primary interest, unlike Charcot's, was in curing the patient, not in amassing a great body of theoretical knowledge. He was both a judicious observer and an alert clinician. By the end of his first four years of work in Nancy, he and his assistants had collected empirical data on five thousand hypnotized cases. In a few more years he had added another five thousand. Even Charcot could not boast such an impressive accumulation of clinical material. And Bernheim raised issue with Charcot: The Salpêtrière, he maintained, overlooked the fact that a great many of the hysterical manifestations they observed had their origin in the hypnotizer's inadvertent suggestions and not in the nature of the disease. Bernheim believed that it was the process of suggestion and the characteristics of suggestibility that should be studied. At length Bernheim's view prevailed. Charcot was unable to disprove his contentions, which were based on a much broader understanding of the problem involved.

Bernheim had thus, starting from the clue Liébeault had given him, broadened the borders of the psychoneuroses to include others besides hysterics. And he had, through his study of suggestibility, made the first historic medical attempt to gain insight into human behaviour in general. Tentative as this attempt was, it was of inestimable value, for it represented the first modern approach to an understanding of human behaviour and its motivation, based not on philosophic presuppositions, but on clinical, empirical observations.

Even though Freud spent only a few weeks at Nancy, the impressions he formed there were soon to lead him out of the static, descriptive maze in which Charcot had left him. For the first time he had seen scientific evidence of a suspicion he had long entertained—"the possibility that there could be powerful mental processes which nevertheless remained hidden from the consciousness of man." A few years later, the recollection of an experiment he had seen Bernheim perform was to make him realize that he could dispense with hypnosis altogether as a therapeutic tool. Thus what he learned at Nancy gave him the final impetus to break completely free of the past, and take off on his own down the lonely road of psychoanalytic exploration.

But he was not quite ready yet to dispense altogether with hypnosis. Back in Vienna, his practice resumed, he tried first the treatment by suggestion in deep hypnosis which he had seen so impressively demonstrated by Liébeault and Bernheim. Although the cures he made were often dramatic, they also tended to be short-lived. While he continued to use the method, *faute de mieux*, he began to suspect that the depth of the cure depended primarily on the personal sympathy between the patient and the physician. With these doubts of the efficacy of suggestion was coupled a feeling of antipathy. He felt the method to be, in a sense, an indignity. At Nancy, along with the pleasure he had felt at the good work accomplished, had come "a feeling of gloomy antagonism against this tyranny of suggestion. When a patient who did not prove to be yielding was shouted at: "What are you doing? *Vous vous contresuggestionez!*" I said to myself that this was an evident injustice and violence."

Meanwhile Bernheim's influence had set him wondering about the question of the origin of his patients' symptoms. He began to see clearly that without understanding the cause of their disorders, he could never hope to devise a really workable method of curing them. In groping for an understanding of this mystery of first causes, certain memories which had long lain dormant floated to the surface of his mind and insisted on being heard. One memory centred about a walk he had taken as a young internee with Dr. Josef Breuer, a well-thought-of Viennese physician whom he had met in Bruecke's laboratory. A man had come up to Breuer on this walk, "and when Breuer was free again," Freud recalled, "he told me in his kindly, teacherlike manner that this was the husband of a patient who had brought some news about her. The wife, he added, behaved in so conspicuous a manner when in company, that she had been turned over to him for treatment as a nervous case. He ended with the remark: 'Those are always secrets of the alcove.' Astonished, I asked him what he meant, and he explained to me the word alcove (conjugal bed), for he did not realize how strange this matter appeared to me."[17]

Another such incident, Freud recalled, had taken place at one of Charcot's evening receptions. Freud had been standing near Charcot, who was describing to a colleague a case that had interested him enormously. The case involved a young married couple. The wife was extremely nervous and the husband either impotent "or exceedingly awkward." Charcot recounted the details of the wife's disturbance. His colleague was astonished that such symptoms as those he described should appear as a result of such circumstances, whereupon Charcot said suddenly and impatiently: "*Mais, dans ces pareils, c'est toujours la chose genitale, toujours—toujours—toujours.*" And while saying that, he had crossed his hands in his lap and jumped up and down several times, with the vivacity peculiar to him. At the time, Freud later said, he was "for a moment . . . almost paralysed with astonishment, and I said to myself, 'Yes, but if he knows this, why does he never say so?' "[18] Although the shock of Charcot's words almost paralysed Freud, the recollection of the incident had been buried in his complete absorption in methods of cure, not causes.

Shortly after this evening at Charcot's, when he had just hung out his plate, and when, he says, he "was as innocent and ignorant in all that concerned the etiology of the neuroses as could only be expected of a promising academician," he received a call from Dr. Chrobak, the gynecologist on the staff of the University. Chrobak was anxious to get rid of a rather tiresome patient, and he was doing

Freud the dubious honour of asking him to treat her. The woman, Freud learned, suffered from senseless attacks of anxiety which could only be relieved if she knew the exact whereabouts of her doctor during every hour of the day. After Chrobak had explained this, his brisk professional manner evaporated. He lowered his voice, took Freud aside and disclosed the fact that the lady's anxiety was undoubtedly due to the fact that she was still a virgin, although she had been married for eighteen years. Her husband was impotent.

"In such cases," said Chrobak, "there is nothing that the physician can do but cover up the domestic misfortune with his reputation, and he must bear it if people shrug their shoulders and say, 'He is not a good doctor if in all these years he has not been able to cure her.' " He added, "The only prescription for such troubles is the one well known to us, but which we cannot prescribe. It is:

Penis normalis
dosim
Repetatur!"[19]

This was the first time Freud had ever heard of such a prescription. He was aghast at what he felt to be his colleague's cynicism. But aghast, startled, shocked or astonished, it was the memory of these incidents that claimed Freud's attention in his inward search for the cause of his patients' neurotic symptoms. Freud's own mind in these early years of his marriage must have been much on matters of sex. That was perhaps one good reason why these memories and these alone proved so obtrusive.

It was Josef Breuer who offered the key which unlocked the mystery, the same man who had spoken so matter-of-factly of the secrets of the alcove. Doctor Breuer was fourteen years older than Freud and one of the most respected family physicians in Vienna. But he was more than that. A man of striking intelligence, he had produced several works of permanent value on the physiology of breathing and on the organ of equilibrium. This work he did in his spare time, generally at night. As a doctor he was held in universal esteem. The great Bruecke himself, his assistants and many other prominent figures in the then world-famous Vienna medical school used him as their personal physician and medical consultant.

With this highly respected member of his own profession Freud had been on increasingly friendly terms since the days when he had first met him in Bruecke's laboratory. "He became," Freud says, "my friend and helper in my difficult circumstances. We grew accustomed to share all our scientific interests with each other. In this relationship the gain was naturally mine." Even before Freud went to Paris, Breuer had told him about a case of hysteria which he had treated, between 1880 and 1882, in a new manner. This method Breuer believed led to a deeper understanding of the cause and significance of hysterical symptoms. Repeatedly Breuer would read to his young friend portions of this case history until Freud became as convinced as Breuer that "it accomplished more towards an understanding of neuroses than any previous observation." In Paris, Freud told Charcot of Breuer's revolutionary treatment, but Charcot, absorbed in his labelling and classifying, showed no interest.

But when Freud began to struggle himself to understand the causes of his patients' behaviour, he returned to Breuer and they picked up the discussion of the ten-year-old case again. The patient, "Anna O.", had been a young and gifted girl. She had become paralytic and mentally confused while she was nursing her father, to whom she was inordinately attached. Breuer had been treating her for some time, when a chance observation showed him that her frequently clouded states of consciousness could be cleared up if she could be made to describe in words the state of mind she was in at the moment. On the basis of the observation, Breuer arrived at a new method of treatment. Each time he saw "Anna O." he would put her into deep hypnosis and make her tell him what it was that was bothering and confusing her. When she awoke her depression and confusion would be gone. He used the same procedure, then, to clear up her physical disorders.

Out of hypnosis, Anna O. had no knowledge of how her

symptoms had arisen, and she could consciously discover no connection between them and any experiences of her life. In hypnosis, she did not hesitate immediately to supply the missing connection. Breuer soon learned that all her symptoms were traceable to emotional upheavals she had experienced while nursing her father. It became apparent that in most instances she had had some thought or impulse while she nursed her father which she had found repugnant and immediately suppressed. In place of the censored impulses, the symptoms had afterwards appeared. As a rule, Breuer found the symptom was not the result of a single such scene, but of a number of similar scenes. When Anna would recall a situation of this kind under hypnosis and reenact with all its attendant emotion the mental act she had originally suppressed, the symptom was magically abolished and did not return. Thus it was apparent that Anna's seemingly irrational hysterical symptoms were eminently meaningful. They were, as Freud says, "residues or reminiscences" of the emotional states she had experienced but never allowed to become conscious.

After long and painstaking effort, Breuer succeeded in relieving Anna of all her symptoms. She had remained well and had even become capable of doing serious work. "But," says Freud, "over the final stage of this hypnotic treatment there rested a veil of obscurity which Breuer never raised for me; and I could not understand why he had so long kept secret what seemed to me an invaluable discovery, instead of making science the richer by it."

Increasingly disaffected with the limitations of treatment by hypnotic suggestion, Freud began to try Breuer's method of probing beneath the patient's conscious mind for a reenactment or catharsis of the emotional disturbances which had caused the symptoms. Soon he abandoned suggestion altogether and for several years used Breuer's method exclusively. He found invariably that what Breuer had done with Anne O. he himself could accomplish with his own hysterical patients. He also found that he could do something Breuer had not done: he could effect a cure through Breuer's "cathartic" method without first putting the patient into a state of deep hypnosis.

This abandonment of hypnosis was forced on him. One day, one of his "most acquiescent patients," upon awakening from hypnotic sleep, threw her arms around Freud's neck. The unexpected entrance of a servant cut short what promised to be a most embarrassing situation. From that time it was tacitly understood between the two of them that there would be no further hypnotic treatment. "I was modest enough," Freud said later on, "not to attribute the event to my own personal attraction, and I felt that I had now grasped the nature of the mysterious element that was at work behind hypnotism. In order to exclude it . . . it was necessary to abandon hypnotism."

It was not the overly affectionate lady alone who convinced Freud that he had better relinquish the two-edged tool of hypnosis. He grew weary with many other patients of hearing, after the command, "You will sleep, sleep now," such protests as, "But, Doctor, I am not sleeping." Freud would then be forced to make a very delicate distinction. He would say, "I do not mean the usual sleep, I mean the hypnotic—you see, you are hypnotized, you cannot open your eyes." or "I really don't want you to sleep." The necessity for all this psycho-semantics confused and embarrased him. He began to feel it would be better to avoid the embarrassment altogether. Whenever his first attempt did not produce either somnambulism or a degree of hypnotism with pronounced bodily changes, he quickly dropped the hypnotic attempt and demanded only "concentration." To help the "concentration" along, he ordered the patient to lie on his back and close his eyes.

Without hypnosis how could Freud expect his patients to reveal the roots of their nervous symptoms in a state which differed only little from their conscious one? Breuer had maintained that it was only in a hypnotic state that such recollections were available. A memory Freud retained from his days at Nancy showed him that he was nevertheless on the right track.

He had seen Bernheim prove that the recollections produced by hypnosis were only manifestly forgotten in the waking state, and that they could readily be reproduced by slight urging accompanied by hand pressure. He recalled the experiment Bernheim had conducted: To a woman in hypnosis he had suggested that he was no longer present in the room. He had then proceeded to make his presence as noticeable as possible, by hitting her, among other things. When she had awakened Bernheim asked her what he had done to her during the time she thought he was not there. She replied in astonishment that he could have done nothing since he was not present. Bernheim insisted that she could recall the truth of the matter if only she tried, and he placed his hand on her forehead as he persisted in the questioning. Freud recalled that she finally related all that she did not apparently perceive in the somnambulic state and about which she ostensibly knew nothing in the waking state.

This instructive experiment became Freud's model. He proceeded on the assumption that his patients were really aware of everything that was of any pathogenic significance, and that all he needed to do was to force them, as Bernheim did, to tell it.

When he reached a point in his treatment where to the question, "Since when have your this symptom?" or "Where does it come from?" he was answered by "I really don't know," he would place his hands on the patients' forehead or take her head between his hands and say, "Under the pressure of my hand it will come into your mind. In the moment that I stop the pressure you will see something before you, or something will pass through your mind which you must note. It is that which we are seeking. Well, what have you seen or what came into your mind?"

When he did this for the first time, he was surprised and pleased to find exactly what he wanted. Gradually he grew bolder. When patients would reply to his insistence, "I see nothing" or "Nothing came into my mind," he told them that that was impossible, that they probably had the right answer but did not believe it and had therefore repudiated it. He found this to be so. The patients would reject the emerging recollection or fancy because they considered it useless, irrelevant or shameful; but after Freud had persuaded them to tell it anyway, he generally found it to be the right one. Sometimes, after he had forced such a confession by pressing the patient's head three or four times, he would be told, "Yes, I was aware of it the first time, but I did not wish to say it," or "I hoped that it would not be this."

With the revision of Breuer's original cathartic method, Freud treated and helped a number of patients with hysterical symptoms. In 1892, a young English governess, "Miss Lucy R.," came to him complaining that she had lost all sensation of smell, save for a persistent odour of burned pastry and cigar smoke which haunted her when there was no burned pastry or cigar smoke about. With his newly revised therapeutic procedure, Freud revealed these symptoms to be—rooted as they were in traumatic events—an hysterical form of defense against her hopeless and consciously unadmitted love for her employer. And he found, as Breuer had with "Anna O.," that when these symptoms were explained, their causes brought into consciousness, and their emotional colour re-experienced, they disappeared.

In the same year he treated another young woman, "Miss Elisabeth v. R.," who after a series of family deaths and misfortunes began to suffer from such acute pains in her legs that she could barely walk. This incapacity Freud traced by the same method to her consciously unrecognized and forbidden love for her brother-in-law.

In whatever hysterical psyche he dug, he seemed always to find at bottom a problem of sex. Freud himself was surprised and even apologetic at the results of his investigations. In the introductory remarks to the book describing his methods, which he and Breuer were soon to publish, he said: "I was not always a psychotherapist, but like other neuropathologists I was educated to the use of focal diagnosis and electrical prognosis, so that even I myself am struck by the fact that the histories of the diseases which I write read like novels and, as it were, dispense with the serious features of the scientific character. Yet I must console myself with the fact that the nature of the subject is apparently more responsible for this issue than my own predilection. Focal diagnosis and electrical reactions are really not important in the study of hysteria, whereas a detailed discussion of the psychic processes, as one is wont to receive it from the poet, and the application of a few psychological formulæ, allows one to gain an insight into the course of events of hysteria."[20]

Breuer was reluctant, despite Freud's urging, to publish their findings. After his first experience with the cathartic method he had forgotten about it, and had only retraced his ten-year-old steps at Freud's insistence. Besides, he had no special interest in the treatment of nervous disorders, and his practice as an internist kept him busy. He objected vehemently to Freud's suggestion that they write a joint paper, but in the end he gave way—principally because, in the meantime, the work of Janet in France had anticipated some of his results. In 1893, Breuer and Freud's first preliminary paper, "On the Psychical Mechanism of Hysterical Phenomena," appeared. It was the first public presentation of the new therapy.

In a scientific era which was in general agreement with Pierre Janet's thesis that hysteria was the manifestation and result of heredity and "degeneracy," this paper stated that "our investigations show that the causes of many, if not of all, cases of hysteria, can be designated as *psychic trauma.* . . . The hysteric suffers mostly from reminiscences." Two years later, Breuer and Freud's book, *Stuedien uber Hysteria,* an expanded and documented version of the preliminary paper, was published. This was an epochal event in the history of medical psychology even if at the time no one thought so. For it made available to the medical world what Freud had known and practised for three years: that the cause of neurotic illness, the symptoms generated by the cause, the therapeutic process revealing and removing the cause were integral parts of a whole. The discovery of this principle, with its attendant implication that there existed an unconscious mind, marked the beginning of a new medical discipline—psychoanalysis.

For the discoveries presented in the *Stuedien* Freud was always careful to give Breuer more than his just share of the credit. For the theoretical contributions presented in the book, which were rudimentary, he held himself partly responsible. Significantly, the *Stuedien* had little to say on the subject of sexuality. And by the time the book appeared, it had become Freud's increasing conviction, based now on what his patients invariably disclosed to him, that disturbances in sexual functioning were root to the diseased plant of neurosis. This estimation of the rôle of sexuality in producing neurotic disorders, which was to become one of the basic planks of the psychoanalytic platform, was then, as it is now, a concept of striking unpopularity. The first one to find it so was Josef Breuer.

There had been differences of opinion between the two men at quite an early stage of their collaboration. But these differences had either been resolved or, without animosity, left unresolved. But when Freud began increasingly to emphasize the significance of sexuality he found "Breuer was the first to show me those reactions of resentful rejection, with which it was my lot to become so familiar later on, but which at that time I had not yet recognized as my inevitable destiny." Soon the collaboration came to an end, and Freud could list Breuer, along with Bruecke and Meynert, in the ranks of his enemies.

Freud wrote those words some fifteen years after his break-up with Breuer. An unmistakably bitter statement, it indicates that even that much later Freud still smarted under what he must have interpreted as Breuer's rejection of him. He had cooled off somewhat by the time he wrote his *Autobiography* in 1925. There he offers a substantially tempered version of the break. In the years following the publication of the *Stuedien,* he says, he read some papers on sexuality and its conditioning rôle in neuroses before various Viennese medical societies, "but was only met with incredulity and contradiction. Breuer did what he could for some time longer to throw the great weight of his personal influence into the scales in my favour, but he effected nothing and it was easy to see that he too shrank from recognizing the sexual etiology of the neuroses. He might have crushed me or at least disconcerted me by pointing to his own first patient, in whose case sexual factors had ostensibly played no part whatever. But he never did so, and I could not understand why this was until I came to interpret the case correctly and to reconstruct from some remarks which he had made the conclusion of his treatment of it. After the work of catharsis had seemed to be completed, the girl had suddenly developed a condition of 'transference love'; he had not connected this with her illness, and had therefore retired in dismay. It was obviously painful for him to be reminded of this apparent contretemps. His attitude towards me oscillated for some time between appreciation and bitter criticism; then accidental difficulties arose, as they never fail to do in a strained situation, and we parted."[21]

Thus the birth and infancy of what Freud was to turn into psychoanalysis were attended by a set of emotional circumstances remarkably similar to those surrounding the infancy of its author. For his work, as for his play with nephew John, Freud had acquired a collaborator superior to him in prestige, as John had been in age and strength. With this collaborator Freud was to repeat the pattern of his childhood relationship.

Freud was always eager to produce the figure of John as a screen, but behind John there lurked the figure of his father, who was cast at an early age in a villainous rôle. It was the father who was really the prototype of all of Freud's later friendly-enemy preceptors. Like the father, Bruecke, Meynert and Breuer were figures of authority who protected and encouraged him in his helplessness. Jacob had not only been a man to look up to and admire. He had also been a stern, commanding voice which in "resentful rejection" ordered him out of his sanctuary; then a voice of anger which told him he would never amount to anything; still later a fallen hero who in meek abjection made way for the insulting Gentile.

His three patrons, Bruecke, Meynert and now Breuer trod the same measures of this "predestined" dance—first venerated; then, once they had voiced disapproval, seen as rejectors; finally, stripped of their heroic robes and rejected in their turn. This "destiny" of Freud's character was, as he said, "inevitable." Hostility towards his father, which he would never permit himself consciously to express, found its outlet in the patrons whom he substituted for his father.

The hostility he felt he projected in carefully general words, after his father's death. Then he wrote: "The authority proper to the father has at an early age evoked the criticism of the child, and the strict demands which he has made have caused the child in self-defense to pay particularly close attention to every weakness of his father's; but the piety with which the father's personality is surrounded in our thoughts, especially after his death, intensifies the censorship which prevents the expression of this criticism from becoming conscious."[22]

That he himself saw an identity between the figures of these protectors and his father is also apparent. After his father's death, he had a dream in which his father appeared in the place of Meynert. The dream took place after he had heard that an older colleague, whose judgment he respected, had expressed shock and disapproval upon hearing that one of Freud's patients had been undergoing psychoanalytic treatment for five years. This colleague, said Freud, probably referring to Breuer, "had for a time taken over the duties which my father could no longer perform . . . ; and when our friendly relations began to alter for the worse I was thrown into the same emotional conflict as that which arises in the case of a misunderstanding between father and son. . . . The dream-thoughts now bitterly resent the reproach that I am not making better progress. . . . The sentence, 'I go to him in the adjoining room' (which appears in the dream) . . . faithfully reproduces the circumstances under which I told my father that I was engaged to be married. Thus the dream is trying to remind me of the noble disinterestedness which the old man showed at that time, and to contrast this with the conduct of another newly introduced person. I now perceive that the dream is allowed to make fun of my father because in the dream-thoughts, in the full recognition of his merits, he is held up as an example to others. . . . The next sentence . . . contains nothing that really relates to my father any more. The person who is screened by him is here a no less important personage than the great Meynert. . . .

"The fact that in this scene of my dream I can use my father to screen Meynert is explained not by any discovered analogy between the two persons, but by the fact that it is the brief but perfectly adequate representation of a conditional sentence in the dream-thoughts which, if fully expanded, would read as follows: 'Of course, if I belonged to the second generation, if I were the son of a professor or a privy councillor, I should have progressed more rapidly.' In my dream I make my father a professor and a privy councillor."[23]

Much of Freud's reason—or compulsion—to split with his patrons emerges in what he says and does not say in discussing this dream. As he implies in his wish for more distinguished parentage, he was disappointed in and perhaps ashamed of his father's low station in life.

Freud was the first to proclaim scientifically that dreams fulfil unrealized wishes, and in his dream he makes his father a professor or a privy councillor. First in his hero-worship, and later in his search for patrons to whom he could cling, he sought unconsciously to replace the father he could take no pride in with a man of prestige and accomplishment. He had been reared in an atmosphere of rigid Jewish piety with the stern necessity to honour his father. Whatever inner recognition of his hostility he allowed himself to admit, outwardly he held steadfastly to the standard which had been set for him. Because he never consciously allowed himself to express any disapproval of his father, his need for revenge for the indignities he felt he had suffered psychologically at his father's hands became intensified, and finally displaced. The emotions he vigilantly dammed up had to break out somewhere.

Moreover, he entertained the fearful unconscious expectation that these men who were his substitute fathers would treat him in the same disapproving way his real father had. Thus, in moving towards them, he moved away from them. In seeking their protection, he expected their disapproval, which he was compelled to interpret—because it was a projection of his own need—as revenge.

This moving toward and away from dependence on a father figure he himself neatly illustrated in a passage he wrote at about this same time which discussed his Parisian day-dreams of finding a protector: "The provoking part of it all," he said, "is the fact that there is scarcely anything to which I am so hostile as the thought of being someone's protégé. What we see of this sort of thing in our country spoils all desire for it, and my character is little suited to the rôle of a protected child. I have always entertained an immense desire to 'be the strong man myself.' "[24]

Despite the immensity of this desire for independence he had by this time successively been the protégé of Bruecke, Meynert and Breuer. It is understandable that his inner struggle should have been projected into his outward life. It is less understandable that the man who was so acute in penetrating the surface of other people's lives should rest content to call it his destiny that he inevitably quarrel with his protectors.

However, from this time on Freud forged straight ahead, whatever disruption and conflict he may have felt inwardly. The uncertainty he had experienced about his choice of a career, and the nature of the contribution he could make within its framework, disappeared.

7

The Stuff of Dreams

Now Freud was free to pursue his own investigations in his own way. He became, as he termed it, the sole administrator of Breuer's legacy. One of the first transformations in the legacy which he effected was a completely new development in the *method* of cure.

As we have seen, when Freud abandoned hypnosis and suggestion, he took to urging his patients somewhat peremptorily, with his hand laid on their foreheads, to tell him the cause of their symptoms. He soon found that trying to force them into revelation was unnecessary and inadvisable. Instead, he proceeded more slowly and indirectly. He would urge them to tell him everything that came to their minds, to omit nothing regardless of whether they considered it unimportant, irrelevant or shameful. He asked them to suspend all critical judgment of what they were saying, to forego all conscious reflection, and to give themselves up to a spontaneous, continuous expression of whatever came into their minds. This process he called "free association."

It was not really free, since the patient remained under the influence of the therapeutic situation. Even though he was not directing his thoughts to a specific subject, Freud found that nothing actually occurred to the patient that did not have some relevance to his basic emotional disturbance. He found, however, that the patient's associations never led him immediately to the root of the matter, but that they flowed and skipped in a seemingly haphazard way around it. Thus the patients, in their elusive fashion, produced material from their lives which alluded to and suggested the nature of their disturbances, without actually letting the cat out of the bag. Freud would listen composedly with rapt attention to the steady stream of associations. He had by this time gained from his substantial experience a general notion of what to expect. He was able either to infer the nature of the unconscious material from the patient's allusions, or he could recognize its general character from the trend of the associations.

Uncovering the root of the patient's disorder by free association, layer by layer, was neither quick nor easy. While free association might seem the long way round of arriving at the same destination, it had definite advantage over the earlier techniques used by Bernheim, Breuer and Freud himself. For one thing, it exposed the patient to the least possible amount of compulsion, the factor of the earlier therapy that had so repelled Freud. For another, it kept Freud in constant touch with the patient's immediate life situation. Freud's part in the process was not that of a listening automaton. To interpret the stream of associations accurately required tact, experience and a kind of intuition difficult to teach to those not naturally gifted with it. Unlike the processes involving hypnotism and forceful urging, the pertinent information made its appearance at various times and at various stages in the treatment.

With the development of the method of free association,* Freud was at last able to document and codify the enormous intuitive insight into human nature which was the natural residue of his own tireless self-searching. Where the methods of suggestion and hypnotism had

* Many years before Freud arrived at the technique of free association, a renowned Swedenborgian and mystic, Dr. Garth Wilkinson, had expounded what he believed to be a new means of literary and religious experience. This was in 1857, and he called his method "Impression." It consisted of first writing down a theme, and then "listening," as Havelock Ellis put it, "to the deepest unconscious expressions from within." Freud undoubtedly knew nothing of Wilkinson's "Impression."

failed to provide him with the answers to the question of why hysterical symptoms appeared and how they developed, the new technique of persuading the patient to reveal and uncover himself from within began almost at once to answer such questions.

Why, for example, had the patient himself invariably forgotten the origins of his symptoms? From the laborious, painstaking culling of his patients' associations, Freud began to reach the conclusion that: "Everything that had been forgotten had in some way or other been painful; it had either been alarming or disagreeable or shameful by the standards of the subject's personality." With this explanation, Freud was well on his way towards the formulation of two of the primary theoretical tenets of psychoanalysis—"resistance" and "repression." Even in the case of ostensibly cooperative patients, there was an inevitable effort to prevent the forgotten material from being uncovered, and this unconscious force, this "resistance," Freud had to overcome. "Repression" was the name Freud gave to the process whereby the patient denied access to the painful impulses and emotions which had set his neurosis in motion.

Once in possession of the theories of resistance and repression,* Freud began to reconstruct their pathogenic process, and he emerged with a blueprint of the motive forces at work in human behaviour that read for all the world like an instruction sheet given out with a complicated machine tool. He spoke of "charges of energy" inherent in instincts or impulses, which were met by the "counter charges" of the neurotic structure. Exact and mechanical, these explanations sound almost like chemical formulæ. Freud's zeal for exact science led him to describe human behaviour in terms of physics. Distorted and dated as these explanations of the dynamics of human behaviour

* "I would very energetically oppose," Freud said early in the history of psychoanalysis, "any attempt to count the principles of repression and resistance as mere assumptions instead of results of psychoanalysis. Such assumptions of a general psychological and biological nature exist . . . but the principle of repression is an acquisition of the psychoanalytic work, won by legitimate means, as a theoretical extract from very numerous experiences."

appear to-day, they nevertheless constitute the first scientific attempt to locate and describe the forces at work in human nature.

The theory of repression* became what Freud called the foundation-stone of his understanding of the neuroses. It led inevitably to the concept of *unconscious* psychic activity which was basic to the new medical discipline he was evolving. Even at this early date he had begun to regard every mental act as having been originally unconscious. The quality of consciousness might also be present, or it might not. But the unconscious was always at work. (For the thinkers of Freud's day, incidentally, the words "conscious" and "mental" were synonymous. An "unconscious" which was also "mental" was an unheard of absurdity.)

Thus, when psychoanalysis was born, it consisted of a new method of treating neurotics, a new clinical way of observing human behaviour, and a new body of theory to explain that perspective. From the first it was more than mere therapy. Its founder had said early in his career that he had no particular enthusiasm for the rôle of physician. And Freud's interest in the new method, even in the earliest days of its life, extended far beyond its therapeutic aspects. At the beginning, when he depended far more on the cumulative clinical evidence of his patients for the development of his theory, he was more interested in theory than in practice. He took pains to hide his preference, for

* The formulation of the theory of repression was worked out independently by Freud. He had long considered the idea to be original until he was shown the passage in *The World as Will and Idea*, in which Schopenhauer tries to explain insanity. "What he [Schopenhauer] states there," Freud said, "concerning the striving against the acceptance of a painful piece of reality agrees so completely with the content of my theory of repression that once again I must be grateful to my not being well read, for the possibility of making a discovery. To be sure, others have read this passage and overlooked it without making this discovery, and perhaps the same would have happened to me if in former years I had taken more pleasure in reading philosophical authors. In later years I denied myself the great pleasure of reading Nietzsche's works, with the conscious motive of not wishing to be hindered in the working out of my psychoanalytic impressions by any preconceived ideas. I have therefore to be prepared—and am so gladly—to renounce all claim to priority in those many cases in which the laborious psychoanalytic investigations can only confirm the insights intuitively won by the philosophers."

he was well aware that the theoretical concepts he was to produce were subject to attack in a mechanist era as "assumptions." Describe them as he might in terms which he regarded as part of an empirical, exact, experimental science, he undoubtedly recognized their closer resemblance to that disreputable vixen—philosophy. This despite his emphatic denials.

Freud was well started by this time on the investigations which were soon to crystallize into one of the most controversial theories he ever sponsored—that neuroses were without exception disturbances of the sexual function. This stand, which he never relinquished, is still hotly debated, attacked and defended by the various schools of psychoanalysis. Some of his earliest conclusions, ones he reached while he and Breuer were still working together, are today naïve. He believed, for example, that various forms of neuroses each showed a different sexual abnormality as their corresponding cause. Anxiety states, he felt, were caused by *coitus interruptus*, undischarged excitement and sexual abstinence. In "neurasthenia," a term which today has little diagnostic meaning, he found excessive masturbation and "too numerous noctural emissions" as the root cause. Where he found a "specially instructive" neurotic who exhibited symptoms of both clinical pictures, he felt that it was possible to show that there had been a corresponding change in the person's sexual habits.

Later observations rang truer. As Freud worked with his patients in these early days of psychoanalysis, he found that his search for the origins of pathogenic situations carried him further and further back into the patients' lives, until finally he ended by reaching the first years of their childhood. The theory of infantile sexuality, even more unacceptable to the world at large than the theory that all neuroses have a sexual origin, did not reach full flower in the first years of tenative analytic investigation. But Freud was being led gradually and inevitably to it as he continued with his archæology of the psyche.

He found, as poets and philosophers had found before him, that the impressions of childhood, although they were for the most part forgotten, had left ineradicable traces upon the individual's development and had in particular laid the foundations of any neurosis that was to follow. But he found, unlike the poets and philosophers, that these childhood experiences invariably revolved around sexual situations, and the reaction against them. Thus he was confronted by the fact of infantile sexuality—once again a new principle which punctured one of the world's most cherished illusions. Childhood, up to Freud's time, had been regarded as "innocent," free from any concern with sex. Puberty had always marked, in the eyes of the world, the first onset of sexual feeling. Sexual activities occasionally observed in children had been ascribed to degeneracy, premature depravity, or freakishness. Few of Freud's findings met with such universal opposition or aroused such outbursts of scorn and indignation as his insistence that the sexual function starts at the beginning of life and betrays its presence by certain signs even in childhood. And yet, Freud felt no other finding of psychoanalysis could be demonstrated so easily and completely.

For a time, Freud was almost thrown off the track of infantile sexuality by an obstacle which he considered to be almost fatal for the young science. He had been accepting as gospel the accounts of patients who traced their symptoms back to seductions experienced in the first years of childhood. His female patients, in order to please Freud or themselves, would almost invariably produce a scene of childhood seduction by their fathers. "If the reader feels inclined to shake his head at my credulity," Freud said ruefully, "I cannot altogether blame him; although I may plead that this was at a time when I was intentionally keeping my critical faculty in abeyance so as to preserve an unprejudiced and receptive attitude towards the many novelties which were coming to my notice every day." When he was forced to recognize the unlikelihood of these tales, for they were easily contradicted by the patient's family, he felt cheated and helpless. Patient after patient whom he treated had invariably revealed such infantile sexual traumas. Yet they were untrue. He began, in despair, to question the validity of his new technique.

Finally he came to the conclusion that no one had a right to despair in the face of one disappointment. (*Man muss ein Stueck Unsicherheit ertragen koennen*, he used to say. "One must learn to put up with some measure of uncertainty.") And he solved the problem to his satisfaction. If his patients persisted in tracing their symptoms back to imaginary, not real sexual experiences, then the neurotic symptoms were not related directly to actual events "but to fantasies embodying wishes, and that as far as the neurosis was concerned, psychical reality was of more importance than material reality." To this thesis the world responded with the charge that Freud had persisted in finding what he looked for; that he had either forced the seduction-fancies upon his patients, or "suggested" them. This he denied. He had in fact gained access for the first time to the road which led him to the Œdipus complex—a concept which he did not yet recognize in its disguise of fantasy, but which was later to assume a central position in psychoanalytic doctrine.

Along with the growth of his conviction that infantile sexuality existed in fact and was revealed in fantasy went his increasing concern with the whole unconscious world of fantasy.

The fact that the apparently nonsensical events of a dream could conceal an eminently rational meaning had come to him as one of the first fruits of free association.* He had not been looking for this discovery. He knew, he said, of no influences which had guided his interest to the intrepretation of dreams. But his work with dreams be-

* Freud states it better. He says: "A dream frequently has the profoundest meaning in the places where it seems most absurd. In all ages those who have had something to say and have been unable to say it without danger to themselves have gladly donned the cap and bells. He for whom the forbidden saying was intended was more likely to tolerate it if he was able to laugh at it and to flatter himself with the comment that what he disliked was obviously absurd. Dreams behave in real life as does the prince in the play, who is obliged to pretend to be a madman; and hence we may say of dreams what Hamlet said of himself, substituting an unintelligible jest for the actual truth: 'I am but mad north-north-west; when the wind is southerly, I know a hawk from a handsaw.' "

came a solace and support to him in those first years of psychoanalysis, when he worked in isolation, difficulty and frequent confusion, and often feared that he would lose both his orientation and his confidence.

Psychoanalytic treatment itself was a long and wearisome process, and Freud must often have doubted the validity of his assumption that a neurosis could be cured by it. But the dreams, which he regarded as similar to symptoms, lent themselves readily to comprehension, and thus gave him hope. His success with dream interpretation, he once said, was the only thing which made him persevere through the difficult years.

There was reason enough for Freud's interest to have taken this turn. Freud himself said in the vast literature of the human spirit he subsequently produced that the most important occurrence in the life of a man was the death of his father. While the father still lived, Freud believed, the son instinctively reacted to him with the full weight of all his historic childish attitudes. In other words, the son remains, at least in relation to his father, a child. When the father dies the physical tie is broken. The son himself becomes a father, whether he has children or not. At this turning-point in life, said Freud, "the tie with the past is broken, and our gaze is henceforward directed towards the future."[25]

For Freud, the death of his father *did* constitute an historic turning-point in his life, and it did, in a sense, liberate him for the full fruition of the work and career he had begun. It was in 1896, when he was forty, that his father died. It was the same year in which he completed in all essentials his original and monumental work, *Die Traumdeutung*, "The Interpretation of Dreams," the first of a long line of contributions to the science of psychology which were to flow from his pen. Later, he found in a book called *Phantasies of a Realist*, by an engineer named J. Popper who wrote under the name of Lynkeus, "the most characteristic and significant portion of my dream theory, namely the reduction of the dream distortion to an inner conflict, to a sort of inner dishonesty. . . ." The connection between *Die Traumdeutung*, which has been called "his greatest single work," and the death of his father has been noted by more than one of his followers. Fritz Wittels, for example, who fell in and out of love with Freud, publicly pointed out in one of his periods of disaffection with his master that Freud's first study with Breuer was published in 1893, a year after the deaths of both Bruecke and Meynert, Freud's scientific fathers. Wittels thought it no accident that this first indication of Freud's entering a new field should follow their deaths. Bruecke and Meynert had both been champions of the organic view of disease. "Not until after their death," Wittels wrote, "could their 'son' openly revolt—not until then could he impulsively turn away from anatomy and physiology." Charcot's death in 1893, according to the *lèse majesté* Wittels later regretted, precipitated Freud into the arms of Breuer, where he remained more or less until the death of his father. Then, says Wittels, "Sigmund grew to full stature and became Freud."

As with so many of the subsequent findings of psychoanalysis, the theories Freud presented in *Die Traumdeutung* as being true of human nature as a whole arose first out of the conditions of his own spirit. On the title page of the book appeared the quotation: *Flectere si nequeo Superos, Acheronta movebo*—literally, "If I cannot influence the celestial Gods, I will set in motion the infernal regions." A freer translation, rendered in the language of Freud's unconscious purpose in writing the book, might read: "If I cannot change my father's attitude towards me, I will let all hell loose." With the publication of the book he did let all hell loose, for his method of interpreting dreams, unlike that of the classic "Egyptian" dream books, laid a well-lighted road into the dark and demented regions of the unconscious mind, whose power he had first recognized in himself. With the conclusions that the book presented, psychoanalysis emerged from being a psychotherapeutic method for the treatment of abnormal conditions, into being a psychology of the depths of human nature, as applicable to the normal mind as to the abnormal. These conclusions were: that the "dream is a psychic act full of import"; that it is an accurate, albeit wilfully distorted mirror of the unconscious life of the mind; that a scientific method of dream interpretation is possible.

Die Traumdeutung led psychoanalysis far from the analytic chamber, into fields of universal interest. Freud himself asserted that his discovery of the meaningfulness of dreams was "a new-found land, which has been reclaimed from the regions of folklore and mysticism." And whether one prefers to believe or not to believe the other thesis which the book presented—that all dreams are the expression of an unfulfilled, unconscious wish—the rest of *Die Traumdeutung*'s findings have become part of the established fact of psychiatry.

The book, when Freud conceived it, was not only a memorial to his father; it was also a coming-of-age gift to himself. For the first time in his career he felt free—or as free as he would ever feel—to reveal himself personally and explicitly. The book provided for Freud the same kind of catharsis his treatment did for his patients. After forty years of living by the dictates of that hard taskmaster—the "immense" desire to be the strong man himself—he was catapulted by his father's death into what amounted to a public confession of his sins. This need to confess and justify himself was a way of explaining himself to his father which he had never felt free to do during his father's lifetime. More than an explanation, the personal testimony in the book constitutes a kind of passionate special pleading to his father for understanding. In the course of the plea, Freud states or implies the whole gamut of emotions intensified by loss and mourning: love and sorrow are evident. Under them, like a subterranean stream, run the currents of revolt, revenge, triumph and self-abasement. Thus *Die Traumdeutung* came to fill a place in his estimation, and incidentally in the estimation of the world, held by no other work of his. "Insight such as this," he wrote about it as late as 1931, "falls to one's lot but once in a lifetime." He felt about it then much as a father does towards a favourite child.

But as the partial, inhibited self-analysis he pursued throughout the pages of *Die Traumdeutung* shows, the leopard cub had not completely changed its spots even in the process of maturing. For all his will finally to psychoanalyse himself, the father of psychoanalysis met within his own psyche a resistance greater than that with which any patient had confronted him. He looked at himself but he did not see himself whole. He still could not bring himself explicitly to identify the nature and content of his hostility towards his father.* He was so intent on justifying himself in the closed eyes of the dead man that resolution of this basic conflict was impossible. He remained, thus, this man who peered so expertly into others' souls, an unsolved mystery to himself. For this reason much of the personal statement he makes is hopelessly contradictory.

For example, in one section of the book he says brusquely: "It is nonsense to be proud of one's ancestors." A few paragraphs later he records the wish that his father might have been a professor or privy councillor—anything, that is to say, of which he might have been proud. And despite his dismissal of pride in ancestry, there runs throughout his self-revelations the theme of his pride in his own children, and his hope that they will be proud of him. At one point the admission is wrung from him that "it is easy to see how the father's suppressed desire for greatness is, in his thoughts, transferred to his children," and he tells us that the wish concealed in the dream he is discussing is "to stand before one's children *great* and *undefiled*." In another dream about a colleague whose career had run parallel to his own for a time until he drew ahead to outstrip Freud both socially and financially, he discovers the meaning of the dream to be his "satisfaction concerning the fact that I have had children by my marriage" while his colleague remained childless.

He is proud of his children. One, he reveals, "is poeti-

* He was, however, aware of the fact that he was repressing some of his feeling. In the interest of discretion, he practically never reported a complete interpretation of one of his dreams. He had what he called "a comprehensible aversion to exposing so many intimate details of one's own psychic life," and he attempted in certain places either to conceal certain details of the meaning of the dream he was discussing or to distort them slightly in order to save himself embarrassment. In spite of his effort towards disfigurement, and the partial nature of his revelation, the main content of his dream emerges clearly enough.

cally gifted." His conversations with his wife, he tells us, sometimes "turned upon the signs of talent which we perceive in our own children." He relates a conversation he once had with a colleague. "How many children have you now?" asked the colleague.

"Six," said Freud.

"A thoughtful and respectful gesture" from the colleague. Then he asked, "Girls, boys?"

"Three of each. They are my pride and my riches," Freud reports himself as having said.

From the weight of the evidence, it appears that despite Freud's own curt decision that pride in one's ancestors is a ridiculous notion, he himself, as a father, expects his children to take quite another view. For, for himself as a father, he believes, "the procreation of children [to be] for all men the only means of access to immortality." And once he awoke from a dream in terror, "even after the idea that perhaps my children will achieve what has been denied to their father [had] forced its way to representation: a fresh allusion to the strange romance in which the identity of a character is preserved through a series of generations covering two thousand years." Thus, on the one hand, he attempts to dismiss his continuity with his father. He scorns the idea of taking pride in him. On the other hand, he is terrified lest the immortality he craves is not sufficiently guaranteed by the six hostages he has created for that purpose.

The information he offers about other aspects of his character is equally contradictory. For example, he says flatly early in *The Interpretation of Dreams,* "I am not, so far as I know, ambitious." Further on in the book he proceeds to analyse a series of dreams which show clearly his great wish to become a full professor—an honour the University never saw fit to confer upon him. He admits his envy of certain colleagues who have been made professors. His preoccupation with his failure to receive a professorship, which he discusses time and again, could only have meant that he craved the prestige which is the fulfillment of ambition. (In *The Psychopathology of Everyday Life,* which he was writing at about the same time *Die Traum-*

deutung was published, he spoke of being lost in an ambitious day-dream which permitted him "to mount always higher and higher.") And finally, despite the disclaimer, he admits his need to excel: "I must always have been ready," he says in interpreting one of his dreams, ". . . to identify myself with Professor R., as this meant the realization of one of the immortal infantile wishes . . . the wish to become great."

The strength of his resistance to revealing himself led him not only into contradictions; it led him into error. In *The Psychopathology of Everyday Life* he discusses some of these errors which he says resulted from repressed thoughts concerning his father. When viewed in the light of Freud's own subsequent discovery that errors, like dreams, are set in motion by the operation of unconscious wishes, the errors he made are extremely revealing. For instance, in naming Hannibal's father in the course of interpreting one of his dreams, he called him Hasdrubal, not Hamilcar Barca, his rightful name. Hasdrubal, as Freud well knew from his long preoccupation with Hannibal, was the name of Hannibal's brother. This error Freud himself attributed to a suppressed fantasy whose content he said was: "How much pleasanter it would be had I been born the son of my brother Emmanuel, instead of the son of my father."

Similarly, he wrote not once but twice in *Die Traumdeutung* that Zeus had emasculated his father Kronos and hurled him from the throne. According to most versions of the myth, it was Kronos who perpetrated this horror on his father Uranos. What Freud did was to advance the crime by a generation. He had made this error, he decided, because of a remark with which Emmanuel had once admonished him. "Do not forget one thing concerning your conduct in life," Emmanuel had said when Freud saw him in England. "You belong not to the second but really to the third generation of your father." Thus Freud implied he had erred because he unconsciously wished to take the job of emasculation of his father upon himself—the third generation, not the second.

Again, in citing the name of Schiller's birthplace, he

made it "Marburg," not "Marbach," which he well knew it should have been. Marburg was a business friend of his father's. The switch of names occurred in the interpretation of a dream which Freud would rather have left in decent mystery; and, indeed, he had tried to veil its meaning. He had broken off the thoughts "which would have contained an unfavourable criticism of my father." But Mr. Marburg, who evoked the memory of an incident in which Freud had been furious with his father, insisted on changing the name of Schiller's birthplace. Thus, the unfavourable criticism of his father, which Freud was trying to keep as much from himself as from his readers, intruded into his consciousness anyway.

Freud was, on the whole, satisfied with the results of his self-analysis. "The analysis of myself," he told a group of American university students in 1909, "the need of which soon became apparent to me, I carried out by the aid of a series of my own dreams which led me through all the happenings of my childhood years. Even today I am of the opinion that in the case of a prolific dreamer and a person not too abnormal, this sort of analysis may be sufficient."[26] Despite Freud's brave avowal, however, it was not sufficient in his case. There was no doctor to psychoanalyse Sigmund Freud. He was the first psychoanalyst, and he was, in the sense that all his theories and discoveries were filtered through his own unconscious mind, his first—and perhaps only—patient. In the usual psychoanalytic relationship between doctor and patient, the patient resists making disclosures to the doctor, and inevitably for a period comes to hate the doctor for forcing him into revealing himself. Freud was doctor and patient at the same time. There was no one for him to resist and vent his hate on except himself. And although he implied to the American students that he had completed his self-analysis, in reality he never stopped eyeing himself. (*"Ich kann mich nicht,"* he said, when he abandoned hypnotism and began to sit behind the patient, seeing him, but not seen himself, *"acht stunden taeglich anstarren lassen."* "I cannot allow myself to be stared at for eight hours a day.") Yet he stared at himself unceasingly for more than half a century, never letting up, never relenting, never ceasing to question his motives or the bases for his judgments. ("*Die Narren*," the fools, Freud once said of his patients. But he knew that he himself was one of his own patients.)

With all the intensive excavation he was to do within his own soul, and with all he accomplished at the time he wrote *The Interpretation of Dreams,* his character, with only minor variations, was to continue to harden in the mould fixed by his original conflicts. He had dared to look at, even if he had not dared to resolve, the hostility and revenge he felt for his father, with the love and reverence which had become intensified by mourning. This division in his emotional life continued. But with his father, that ambivalent object of affection, gone, it changed its direction and it changed its goal.

His repressed rejection of his father became, at this turning-point of his life, a pervasive kind of rejection, sharp, severe and obstinate, aimed against any attempt to solve a problem by appeal to an authority. With the zeal of a convert, he carried this attitude to a fanatic pitch. He not only would make no concession to authority, tradition or prejudice, but he would make no concession to his own frailties, his own wishes and weaknesses. He was equally scornful of weakness in others. He had hardened himself at great pain and cost to the likeness of a fine precision instrument. For half-measures, for weakness, for failures to fulfill duty, he had little sympathy. Hanns Sachs saw him once when Freud had just learned that an old friend had committed suicide. Sachs found him "strangely unmoved" by such a tragic event. For suicide in general meant to him the shirking of a task, an evasion of responsibility. Hard as a scalpel, he would neither express nor give sentimentality. Social conventions, whose expediency he recognized, he rebelled against, for he took no joy in social situations. He remained nevertheless, without any trace of softness, an essentially kind man; and with little evidence of compassion, a benevolent one.

Perhaps more than any other single change that came over him at this, the half-way mark of his life, was the crystallization of his intellectual resolution and purpose. Having examined himself as mercilessly as he could, he seems to have forsworn all the gayer, lighter, softer aspects of life. It might almost be said that he consciously eradicated from his life most of the emotions and occupations which ordinarily make for joy. He began to regard life as an obligation that had been imposed upon him, as a duty which he must fulfil. From this time on, his life was to be his work. His work was to be a relentless search for truth as absolute as he could find it. Neither the impossibility of finding such truth nor the opposition of the world was to deflect him. For this stern purpose he arrayed himself psychically, with the independence, courage and pride that had always been hallmarks of his character, in the armour of siege.

He resembled in these first years of psychoanalysis' development a man who stands alone before an impregnable fortress which he wishes to storm, armed only with an idea. The idea happened to become one of those few which moved the world. At the time, however, Freud, if he was considered at all, was regarded as a crackpot.

The years between 1896, when his father died, and 1898 were the most productive of his life. The discoveries in these few years were truly astounding. As one of his disciples was later to put it, this was a "period of such intense mental activity as is seldom vouchsafed to any man." To these years belong not only the beginnings of the therapeutic technique of psychoanalysis, but *The Interpretation of Dreams*. In addition, he had formulated the theories of resistance and repression. He had traced, in *The Psychopathology of Everyday Life*, the effect of repression on memory and its meaning for the phenomenon of everyday forgetfulness. He had made the first tentative formulation of the sexual theory of neuroses, and had claimed the existence of infantile sexuality. He had intimated that the Œdipus complex existed—it was mentioned for the first time in *The Interpretation of Dreams*.* He had already

* These are the words whose sound has now reverberated around the world. "If the *Œdipus Rex* is capable of moving a modern reader or playgoer no less powerfully than it moved the contemporary

begun to revise the psychoanalytic technique with tools which still serve to-day. The substance of psychoanalysis, in other words, already existed in perfect miniature of what it was later to become.

In spite of the magnitude of these discoveries, any one of which should have been sufficient to bring him fame, he stood at the turn of the century alone and unhonoured. The rejection which he had felt in the days of his unsureness continued now to dog the years of his maturity. In the right little, tight little world of Viennese medicine, he and his new disciples were regarded, if they were honoured by any regard at all, either with contempt or condescension. Freud has said of these years that he unhesitatingly sacrificed his growing popularity and practice in nervous diseases because of his insistent probing for the sexual origin of his patients' neuroses. He had hoped to be compensated for this loss by the interest and recognition of his colleagues. But one appearance as a speaker at the Vienna Neurological Society, then under the presidency of Krafft-Ebing, showed him his error. Silence followed his lecture. Insinuations were directed against him. A void formed about him. He was forced to realize that while he could treat his discoveries as ordinary contributions to science, his colleagues were incapable of viewing his statements about sex in this light. It was also apparent that the élite members of the Neurological Society were not prepared to shout hosannas for a Jew. And it is more than

---

Greeks, the only possible explanation is that the effect of the Greek tragedy does not depend upon the conflict between fate and human will, but upon the peculiar nature of the material by which this conflict is revealed. There must be a voice within us which is prepared to acknowledge the compelling power of fate in the *Œdipus*, while we are able to condemn the situations occurring in . . . other tragedies of fate as arbitrary inventions. And there actually is a motive in the story of King Œdipus which explains the verdict of this inner voice. His fate moves us only because it might have been our own, because the oracle laid upon us before our birth the very course which rested upon him. It may be that we were all destined to direct our first sexual impulses towards our mothers, and our first impulses of hatred and violence towards our fathers. Our dreams convince us that we were. King Œdipus, who slew his father Laius and wedded his mother Jocasta, is nothing more or less than a wish-fulfilment—the fulfillment of the wish of our childhood."[27]

likely that they were repelled by the stiff-necked pride and obduracy with which Freud presented his theories.

For Freud, the feeling of being shunned was not new. He comforted himself in typical fashion—with the characteristic withdrawal of the Jew into hurt pride intensified by the hurt. He reasoned that from that time on he belonged with those who "have disturbed the world's sleep" and that therefore it was unreasonable for him to expect either tolerance, sympathy or objectivity. He was, he later said, "imbued with the conviction that it fell to my lot to discover particularly important connections, and was prepared to accept the fate which sometimes accompanies such discoveries."

This fate he pictured to himself in the bleakest possible colours: "I should probably succeed," he thought, "in sustaining myself through the therapeutic successes of the new procedure, but science would take no notice of me during my lifetime. Some decades later, someone would surely stumble upon the same, not untimely things, compel their recognition and thus bring me to honour as a forerunner whose misfortune was inevitable. Meanwhile, I arrayed myself as comfortably as possible like Robinson Crusoe on my lonely island."[28]

For this "splendid isolation," which he had first encountered in his university days, he was quick with wounded pride to find compensation. He began to see advantages and even charm in what he characterized in retrospect as this "beautiful and heroic era." He was left strictly alone, and so was subject neither to influences nor to pressure. In his isolation, he would often recall Charcot's advice, and look at the same things again and again until they themselves, he said, "began to talk to me." He did not have to read, he reflected with wry irony, any of the medical literature or listen to any ill-informed opponents. His books and articles, for which he could with difficulty still find a publisher, could safely remain far behind the state of his knowledge, since they were hardly read in any case. They could be and were postponed as long as he pleased while in his mind's eye he brought them to a perfect pitch of exact formulation. *The Interpretation of Dreams,* for example, he had formulated completely by the beginning of 1896. But he did not bother to write it down until the summer of 1898. And it was not published until 1900. The case of "Dora," a paper in which he discussed the technical phenomenon of "transference" which was to become a vital part of the therapeutic technique, he wrote in 1899, but did not publish until six years later. He could thus polish, formulate and recollect in complete trănquillity.

There was a further advantage, as he saw it, to his isolation and uninterrupted immersion in psychoanalysis. He interpreted his rejection by the outside world in psychoanalytic terms. (He was, incidentally, also engaged at this time in interpreting his friends psychoanalytically—inferring, from unconscious signs which they gave, nefarious conclusions about the character of their mutual relationship. One friend, incensed by this procedure, bade Freud sharply to leave off treating his friends. Freud, in all humility, agreed with the wisdom of this injunction.) From the fact that his patients met him with inner emotional resistance, he deduced that normal people would also resist the bringing to light of uncomfortable knowledge. And the fact that these normal people, his opponents, resisted him on intellectual grounds did not trouble Freud for a moment. He had met this same phenomenon in his patients who advanced similar arguments. Solaced by his superior knowledge of his opponents' motives in rejecting him and his discipline, Freud says that he was saved from becoming embittered—a statement which resembles a wish-fulfilment more closely than a fact.

Whether he was unembittered or not, the superiority in which he clothed himself helped maintain his resolution to appear unmoved by the criticism of his colleagues, who had dismissed *Die Traumdeutung* with ridicule, and who used in their rare references to his work such adjectives as "unbalanced," "extreme," or "very odd." And he was able to extract a certain acrid amusement out of incidents such as this: A medical novice asked permission to attend some of Freud's lectures, to which he listened attentively. After the last lecture, he asked Freud's permission to accompany him home, and during the course of this walk he told him that he had already written a book attacking Freud's theories, but that after having listened to Freud expound his viewpoint, he now regretted it very much. He had, before writing the book, inquired of his superiors whether it would be advisable to read *The Interpretation of Dreams*, but he had been told not to bother, since it was not worth the trouble. This neglect he now too regretted, since, he told Freud, he had come to regard the solidity of Freud's theoretical structure with that of the Catholic Church, a remark which must certainly have given pause even to Freud. But he wound up by saying that it was too late to rectify his error; the book was already in the process of publication. Nor later, when this man became a permanent reviewer on the staff of a medical journal, did he ever admit that he had been favourably impressed by psychoanalysis. On the contrary, he continued to report its development by making fun of it.

"Whatever personal sensitiveness I possessed," Freud later said, "was blunted in those years—to my advantage." And he added, "That I have not developed any particular respect for the opinion of the world or any desire for intellectual compliance during those years when I alone represented psychoanalysis, will surprise no one."[29] For Freud stood at the turn of the century, when *The Interpretation of Dreams* was published, in a position remarkably similar to the one he had placed himself in when his father had angrily remarked that he would never amount to anything. Not his father this time, but the whole world of medical authority about him said in effect, when he presented them with his accomplishment: "This boy will never amount to anything." His answer to this was the same as his unconscious answer to his father had been: he would show them anyway. But this time his "showing them" took on a different cast. With the knowledge and conviction of his own abilities and achievements strong within him, his self-vindication became almost Messianic.

It is doubtful whether anyone feels himself a Messiah who has not been sufficiently provoked by furious opposition to his ideas to an intensity of belief in himself equal and opposite to the lack of belief which greets him. This was the case with Freud. The opposition which greeted him in these early days grew in force as psychoanalysis developed, until it reached a pitch which must have seemed almost insane to him. Perhaps other men, with characters less attuned to the sounds of rejection, real or imaginary, could have thrown off more easily the insults of their tormentors. But Freud had been quick, before the tumult and the shouting against him had really had a chance to gather its strength, to see himself as Robinson Crusoe, alone except for his resourcefulness, on a desert island. He had been quick to see a wholesale and thoroughgoing humiliation before it actually was put upon him, not only because of his father, but because he was a Jew. As a Jew he had not only met with discrimination, but he expected to find it before he heard its first cawing notes.

As a matter of fact, Freud once in an unguarded moment acknowledged the fact that it was "perhaps no mere chance that the first psychoanalyst was a Jew." For the Jew, driven inward by his sense of segregation from the outside world, turns back upon himself and builds an inner world in which he finds comfort, courage and heroism. Centuries of persecution and isolation have taught the Jew a deep knowledge of man at his worst, and have given him the clue of recognition of man at his best. From this knowledge, which Freud perhaps of all Jews best personified, and from his own inner world of dreamed-of glories and dreamed-of vindication, Freud spun the stuff of which psychoanalysis was made. Almost one might say that, instead of the Judaism he had been born into, a religion he unconsciously resented because it had forced upon him the isolation which, "splendid" as it might be construed to be, still hurt, he had constructed for himself the substitute religion of psychoanalysis.

8

See How It Grows

In retrospect, Freud remembered his period of isolation as having been longer than it really was. Actually, by 1902, a small group of doctors, writers and æsthetes had begun to gather around him. "The impetus for this," Freud says, "came from a colleague who had himself experienced the beneficial effects of the analytic therapy." At first the group numbered only Alfred Adler, tiny, poised, contained at times, excitable at others; Wilhelm Stekel, who was later to publish an important work on dream symbolism; Max Kahane, an old friend of Freud's who had translated Charcot and Janet into German and who was to break with Freud before many years had passed; and Rudolf Reitler. Before long, the circle was joined by Paul Federn, Eduard Hitschmann, Max Steiner and Isidor Sadger, all of whom became practising psychoanalysts. Occasionally Max Graf and David Bach, Vienna's well-known music critics, would sit in on the meetings, as would Friedjung, the specialist in children's diseases, and Hugo Heller, the bookseller. Fritz Wittels joined the group, and also a young graduate of the technical school, Otto Rank, who showed them a manuscript which Freud thought unusually promising, and which caused Freud to persuade him to go through the University with an eye towards devoting himself to the nonmedical application of psychoanalysis. The little circle gained in Rank an eager and conscientious secretary, and Freud a faithful helper and collaborator.

While this group with its protean composition began to meet weekly to study the new doctrine from the lips of its discoverer, the rest of Vienna persisted in ignoring Freud or in treating him as a butt. In those days, Max Graf recalled, when Freud's name was mentioned in a Viennese gathering, everyone would begin to laugh as if someone had made a joke. It was considered bad taste in polite circles even to mention Freud's name in the presence of ladies. If this gaffe were committed, the ladies would blush and titter just as they might at an off-colour story.

In the world of Viennese medicine and in official academic circles, Freud was also considered a bad joke. Although he had been given the title of "professor extraordinary" at the University in recognition of his earlier work in neurology, this was a far cry from a regular professorship; and the time assigned him to deliver his lectures—Saturday evenings from seven to nine—was not calculated to attract large audiences. Wagner von Jauregg, a leading figure in the Viennese medical world, and the regular University professor of psychiatry, headed the medical opposition to Freud. Slow, heavy and taciturn, he was constitutionally incapable of understanding Freud's ideas. He believed the body to be the only concern of medical science. (It was he, incidentally, who discovered the treatment of general paralysis with malaria, one of the great creative discoveries of modern medicine.) Freud and he had been medical students together, and while their surface relationship was politely correct, they were bitter opponents, representing as they did the two opposite poles of psychiatric investigation.

Wagner-Jauregg, like the rest of Vienna, was fond of combating psychoanalysis with ridicule. Psychiatrists, he would tell his pupils, were either "born" or "accidental." He knew of only two "accidental" ones—himself and a colleague. All the others, and by these he meant the upstarts of Freud's persuasion, were "born"—that is to say, they were inevitably attracted to psychiatry because of their own abnormality.

It was in the lecture hall of the Psychiatric Clinic attached to the *Allgemeine Krankenhaus*, the auditorium regularly given over to the lectures of the hostile Wagner-Jauregg, that Freud began at the turn of the century to deliver his Saturday evening lectures. The auditorium, adjacent to the *Narrenturm* or "Fools' Tower," in which the insane had been kept chained to the walls until the beginning of the nineteenth century, was lit on the occasion of Freud's lectures only by a few dim bulbs above the podium. The rows of benches, well filled for the popular Wagner-Jauregg, stretched in empty ascent to meet the ceiling. In the large, dim room, the six or seven psychoanalytic disciples, nearly all of whom were also members of the weekly circle, would huddle together in a semicircle close to Freud's table. Despite the sea of empty space that stretched around them, Hanns Sachs at least found the atmosphere intimate and informal.

Sachs, who first came to one of the lectures in 1904, moved by a need for more of the "stupendous revelations" he had found in *Die Traumdeutung*, found Freud a "middle-aged gentleman who wore a short dark-brown beard, slender and of medium size. He had deep-set and piercing eyes and a finely shaped forehead, remarkably high at the temples." Other members of Freud's circle saw him differently at the same time. Max Graf found that "the very black hair of his head and beard had begun to show traces of grey. The most striking thing about him was his expression." His beautiful, serious eyes "seemed to look at man from the depths. There was then something distrustful in this look; later there was to appear bitterness as well. Freud's head had something artistic about it; it was the head of a man of imagination." Wittels was impressed with his youthful vigour, although Freud was approaching fifty. His eyes, Wittels found, were *not* large and piercing, but "dark brown, lustrous, scrutinizing." His movements were brisk and his slender form was bent in a student's stoop. Hitschmann saw Freud as looking "artless, not striking like other intellectuals or doctors; in a well-fitting suit of fine quality, always with a black tie—he seemed not to have wasted much time on his appearance."

At these lectures, Freud often spoke without notes for nearly the whole two-hour period. The tone and manner of his talks were simple and conversational although the subject-matter, the theory and technique of psychoanalysis, was not. Sachs marvelled at the amazing effect Freud's lectures produced, and decided that the effect lay in their contrast. He had a way of leading to a startlingly original line of thought so gradually and logically that his listeners found themselves carried along on an inevitable swell of reason. He would begin by stating the necessary, essential facts and basic principles with equal caution. He would then detour to discuss all possible objections which might be raised before he discussed his conclusions at length. Then when he took off again on the road to original discovery, it seemed to those listeners of his the most natural thing in the world. "In this way," said Sachs, "he led his hearers insensibly on, never giving them the impression that they were participating in a difficult and quite original investigation. They were surprised when they arrived in the end, without mental gymnastics or contortions, at results that contrasted strangely with some of their previously most cherished opinions or prejudices."[30]

The subjects of the lectures ranged from dream interpretation, the unconscious, repression, and the structure of neurosis, to some of the possible applications of the new science to other fields of knowledge.

After the lectures, the whole group, elated by a sense of high intellectual adventure, used to accompany Freud through the long courtyards of the *Krankenhaus* as far as the *Alser Strasse*. There Freud would leave to take a cab home, where he would meet his old friends Professor Koenigstein, Dr. Rie and Herr Frankfurter, the chief librarian at the University, for the weekly session of the traditional card game of Vienna, *tarock*, which was virtually the only social diversion he permitted himself. Like everything else in his life, this card game followed certain well-established patterns and customs. It was held invariably on Saturday nights and it was played for decades with the same three old friends. In fact, when Koenigstein, the same ophthalmologist to whom Freud had first suggested the use of cocaine, died, he was replaced in the game by another Koenigstein. Even at cards, which he thoroughly enjoyed, Freud's analytic eye pierced beneath the surface experience to find out why the game was pleasurable. He discovered that "when free sway is given to avaricious intent outside of the serious interests of life, when it is indulged in in the spirit of fun, as in card-playing, we then find that the most honourable men show an inclination to errors, mistakes in memory and accounts, and without realizing how, they even find themselves involved in small frauds. Such liberties depend in no small part also on the psychically refreshing character of the play. The saying that in play we can learn a person's character may be admitted if we can add 'his repressed character.' "[31]

The little band of devout psychoanalytic disciples met weekly at Freud's house at Berggasse 19, to which he had long since moved from the "House of Atonement," and in which he was to continue to live until he was forced to flee Vienna. Traditionally, Viennese doctors established their consulting-rooms in their homes, and Freud was no exception. The small, quiet house in which he lived for nearly half a century stood in a district of Vienna popularly known as the "Nobelghetto." The Danube Canal which runs through the district separates the *Berggasse* section from the Ghetto proper. Freud's district was predominantly populated by Jews of the middle class.

Berggasse, true to its name, is a steeply rising street, even for the hilly terrain of Vienna. It starts at the Tandelmarkt, Vienna's ancient junk market, and winds up at the Votivkirche, a modern Gothic cathedral which dominates an ornamental square close to the University, just as the church of St. Mary's Birth dominated the Square of Freiberg. Freud's house was closer to the disreputable world of the junk market than it was to the respectable world of the cathedral and University, but the neighbourhood was quiet and orderly—if undistinguished. A wide stone flight of stairs flanked by a balustrade curved up to two doors on the landing, the one on the right for Freud's patients, the left-hand one for the family's use. Soon a butcher's shop would occupy the street level space.

At first Freud's consulting-room had been on the first floor and his living quarters on the second. But after some years he moved his consulting-room to the second floor, and the family of nine crowded into the five rooms or so of the ground floor. The house, living and working quarters, was furnished in the style and taste of middle-class Viennese homes of the 'eighties. The second-floor suite, which was sacred to Freud's use, consisted of a dark little ante-room and three larger rooms—waiting-room, consulting-room, and *sanctum sanctorum*—the study-library which connected with the consulting-room. None of these rooms was either light or sunny. Each had only one window opening on a bare courtyard in the centre of which a tall tree grew in solitary splendour. Freud scorned ostentation in much the same way he scorned weakness. While his home was comfortable, it was extremely modest.

The little ante-room was bare save for a row of pegs, like those in a schoolroom, where patients' coats were hung. The waiting-room was small and so poorly heated that one visitor felt as if "the best of associations could be frozen in only a few minutes." On the waiting-room table lay the doctor's usual assortment of ancient, tattered magazines—seldom replenished. A small bookcase contained only a collection of gift volumes Freud had not thought sufficiently well of to include in his own library. A large Etruscan vase stood against one wall. In the consulting-room, whose walls were decorated with figures of Egyptian priests, an old-fashioned porcelain stove stood edgewise in a corner. It heated the room, but it gave off an odour which merged with the general airlessness, the musty leather of the book bindings and the hard, dusty odour of the horse-hair sofa with its elevated headpiece on which the patients lay.

Back through a wide, doorless opening, flanked by cabinets which contained Freud's budding collection of ancient *objets d'art,* stretched his long, narrow study, the one room of the suite that bespoke the man. Here, close to the window through which the lone tree peered, stood the Professor's desk, comfortably littered with papers, ivory figurines, ancient relics and a large, circular ash-tray, on which rested his inevitable cigar.

The walls of the study were covered with bookcases which reached nearly to the ceiling. It was in this room, concentrated under a cloud of cigar smoke, that Freud worked alone every evening save Wednesday and Saturday until long past midnight.

In the offices at Berggasse 19 the little group of analytic devotees met, beginning in 1902, each Wednesday evening. Most of them were prepared to participate wholeheartedly in the solemn spirit of high purpose that permeated the musty air of the suite. Everything in the rooms seemed important to them, for the house was, as far as they were concerned, the shrine not of a science but of a cause. The couch and the armchair behind it in the consulting-room might well have been the throne and cross of the Lord for the awe in which they were held. For most of this early group recognized in these meetings, as Max Graf did, "an atmosphere of the foundation of a religion," with Freud as its new prophet and themselves as its new apostles.

Just as Christ's disciples were ranged round their Master in the order of their merit, so this early Freudian group took their places around the long table in the waiting-room according to the estimation in which Freud held each of them. At the beginning Adler and Stekel were the reigning favourites, and to them were accorded the places of honour to the right and left of the master, respectively. Ritual was established. The order in which the members of the group were permitted to speak during the discussion period was decided by lot. Rank, who acted as secretary, arranged the drawing of the lots.

Freud would take the chair at the head of the table. He was almost invisible in the cloud of cigar smoke that hung over him. Before the business of the meeting began, refreshments were served. All partook as if it were wine and wafers, not black coffee and cigars.

Business began with the reading of a paper which bore either directly or indirectly on psychoanalysis. Freud would take up his part of the evening in a manner far bolder than that of his public lectures. First he would state his main line of argument categorically. Then he would offer such an overwhelming wealth of evidence in support of his thesis that none of his listeners could fail to be convinced of its truth. He spoke emphatically, but he spoke quietly, rarely raising his voice at all. He used no oratorical tricks. He spoke at these meetings as he spoke all his life, with the imagination of an artist, the erudition of a scholar, the fervour of a devout believer. For this speech there was no rebuttal. The last, decisive word was reserved for him alone. When he was finished, discussion, in which he expected everyone to participate, was in order.

Certainly the spirit which was to move Freud in his guidance and development of the infant science for the rest of the years of his life would bear out this appearance of ritual and religion. He came to act as if he walked intuitively but no less certainly in the path of his ancestors and in the belief of one of the oldest Jewish traditions—the tradition that all Jews were present on Mount Sinai and there took upon themselves "the yoke of the Law." This yoke rested particularly heavy on Freud. It became a mission, Messianic in character. His psychoanalytic discoveries were to become in his mind and that of some of his devout followers a body of Law as world-shaking and divinely inspired as any ever promulgated by Moses or Jesus. The dissemination of the psychoanalytic doctrine Freud was to handle in the manner of a high priest and prophet dedicated to the missionary task of spreading the gospel.

For the job of spiritual head of his new religion, Freud borrowed some of the characteristics of the God of the Jews—the angry, vengeful Jehovah under whose dominion he had been born. Like Jehovah, Freud created a climate of uneasy reverence among his psychoanalytic acolytes. He became, for all of them who could stand his zealotry, the father, the hope and the hero. They, too, came, through the spiritual atmosphere Freud generated, to regard psychoanalysis as a new religion.

The new religion, under Freud's leadership, was to grow at the beginning in much the same way as other religions have. It, too, was based on an act of faith—only this time the faith was called "scientific rationalism." It, too, was marked by a hierarchy of apostles, by the trappings, schisms and dogma characteristic of the founding of most religions. There were to be faithful disciples like Abraham, Eitingon, Jones, Ferenczi and Sachs, who never took the name of their god in vain and who never bowed down before any graven image; and there were to be "Judases" like Jung, Adler and others who were regarded as dangerous heretics by the small band of the faithful, and finally excommunicated. There was to be an international psychoanalytic organization whose function, like that of any religious missionary organization, was to spread enlightenment among the ignorant. There was to be devotion to every spoken and written word of the master, and a kind of inbred preoccupation with interpreting and defending the dogma rivalled only by the intellectual pursuits of the Talmudists.

"Sigmund," as his disciple Wittels, who was both attracted and repelled by this atmosphere, had so aptly put it, had indeed grown "to full stature and become Freud."

United as the group appeared to be, even at this early date some of its members were repelled by Freud's autocratic control of the whole procedure. To one of them, the ordained rôles assigned to each participant produced an inevitable monotony. To him it seemed that the only purpose of the meetings in Freud's eyes was to have his own ideas thrown back to him by a room full of sounding-boards. It did not matter to Freud at all, he thought, what quality of sounding-boards were present. On the contrary, Freud was better pleased with those members of the group who were neither critical, original, nor ambitious. Fritz Wittels, in particular, felt this keenly. He concluded from repeated attendance at the meetings that "the realm of psychoanalysis was his [Freud's] idea and his will, and he welcomed anyone who accepted his views. What he wanted was to look into a kaleidoscope lined with mirrors that would multiply the images he introduced into it."

Wittels could not bear the position to which he found himself relegated by Freud. Neither could Max Graf, the talented music critic. Wittels thought that Freud's manner of stating his views was so unrelenting it was "apt to repel." He saw members of the group as "adversaries" of Freud, whom the master "overthrew" by reason of the superior force of his arguments. Wittels was not the only member of the group who felt, despite his admiration and respect for Freud, a conflicting current of opposition. Besides Wittels, who eventually left the fold only to return later, Adler, Stekel, Rank and Graf, among these earliest analytic *aficionados*, were in short order to cast off the binding robes of the diciples.

Graf was as divided in his feeling for Freud as Wittels. He found Freud to be endowed with a great "human simplicity" and an absence of any vanity in his scientific personality. But he thought, on the other hand, that Freud was serious and strict in the demands he made on his pupils, that "he permitted no deviation from his orthodox teaching." Freud, nearing fifty, had carried a rocking-horse up four flights of stairs to present to Graf's three-year-old son on his birthday. So Graf knew him to be as good-hearted and thoughtful in his personal friendship as he was hard and relentless in the presentation of his ideas. "When his psychoanalysis was attacked," Graf later said, "he would break with his most intimate and reliable friends." Finally and despairingly, Graf concluded that there was only one way left for him to maintain his self-respect. Unable and unwilling "to submit to Freud's 'do' or 'don't' . . . nothing was left for me but to withdraw from the circle," he said. But even in the act of withdrawing, Graf looked back regretfully, uncertain whether he had not after all been too harsh in his judgment. "If we do consider him [Freud] as a founder of a religion," he said, then it would be reasonable for Freud to act with the complete assumption of authority he had. He saw Freud "as a Moses full of wrath and unmoved by prayers—a Moses like the one Michelangelo made of stone—in the church of San Pietro in Vincoli in Rome."[32] With this identification with Moses, Freud himself was later to agree.

Freud's own opinion of the Wednesday evening meetings and of the reason for their dissolution was entirely different from those of his disaffected followers.

"From the very beginning," Freud said in 1909, "our circle included those men who later were to play a considerable, if not always an agreeable, part in the history of the psychoanalytic movement. But these developments could not be imagined at that time. I was satisfied and I believe I did all I could to convey to the others what I knew and had experienced. There were only two inauspicious circumstances which at last estranged me inwardly from this circle. I could not succeed in establishing among the members that friendly relation which should obtain among men doing the same difficult work, nor could I crush out the quarrels about the priority of discoveries, for which there were ample opportunities under these conditions of working in common. The difficulties of teaching the practice of psychoanalysis, which are particularly great, and are often to blame for the present dissension among psychoanalysts, already made themselves felt in this Viennese private psychoanalytic society. *I, myself did not venture to present an as yet incomplete technique, or a theory which was still in the making, with that authority which might have spared the others many a pitfall and ultimate derailment.** The self-reliance of mental workers, their early independence of the teacher, is always gratifying psychologically, but a scientific gain only results when certain, not too frequently occurring, personal conditions are also fulfilled in the workers. For psychoanalysis in particular a long and severe discipline and training in self-control is really necessary. In view of the courage displayed by devotion to a subject so ridiculed and poor in prospects, I was disposed to tolerate among the members much to which I would otherwise have objected."[33]

It is quite evident from Freud's words that he had no great respect for these earliest of his followers. As an old man, he said in private conversation that he was forced to make the best of the co-workers available to him at the time. He knew when they first appeared on his horizon

* Italics mine.

that they had been drawn to him not so much because of their abstract interest in psychoanalysis, but because of their personal need. He damns them with faint praise: "Our circle," he said, "was hardly inferior to the staff of any clinical teacher." He could find much in them to object to, but he would tolerate them.

In reality, Freud's attitude when his first disciples appeared was much more than just toleration. To him they represented the rescuers who would take him off his lonely island where he lived as proudly and self-sufficiently as Robinson Crusoe, to be sure, but bereft of human company. Those believers not only comforted Freud in his scientific isolation. They were an instrument of hope—hope that his message would be learned and spread.

But he hoped for too much. He came to regard these men, despite his clear recognition of their limitations, as his spiritual sons who would insure his scientific immortality in the same way that his real sons would provide for his physical immortality. It was his paternal attitude, combined with his conviction of his destiny, that established the climate for all the conflicts, schisms and quarrels that were soon to beset him and his infant science. To these children of psychoanalysis he became the kind of father he had known best—rigid, authoritarian, impatient with any deviation from the path of the paternal will. He had outgrown his immature need for dependence. But in the *volte-face* he had performed, he had assumed the face his father had worn for him.

So, while the father of the psychoanalytic movement felt that the authority he brought to bear was not sufficient, the testimony of the psychoanalytic sessionists leads us to believe the reverse.

There are external facts, of course, which can be offered in extenuation of Freud's attitude. It is true, for example, that psychoanalysis requires a broader, more amorphous, and more peculiarly personal aptitude on the part of its practitioners than other fields of scientific endeavour. It is also true that the training is arduous and specialized. And as Freud recognized, because his theories struck at people's emotional security everywhere, his fate would be one of rejection, ridicule and indignity. Yet, even given these circumstances, if Freud had not been impelled by an inner necessity to treat the secular growth of his discovery as an adjunct of his own personality, the external history of the psychoanalytic movement would never have taken the schismatic, cultist course it did.

The relationship between Hanns Sachs and Freud perhaps best illustrates the results of Freud's attitude. Sachs knew Freud for more than thirty years. He was, during this period, first a member of his audience at the Psychiatric Clinic, then a disciple, then a member of the circle of his intimates, and a regular guest in his house, and finally his collaborator and companion. For Sachs, Freud was "the great event and adventure of my life." But Sachs, towards the end of his life, felt impelled to make a confession: Freud, he believed, did not find in him those qualities which he valued most highly. The "something" that leads to warm-hearted intimacy between friends and equals engaged in the same work was missing. It was not the difference in their intellectual statures. Nor was it the gulf that separates the genius from the non-genius. Nor was it anything that Sachs had done that stood between them. For . . . "only once," Sachs wrote as a once naughty, now repentant child might have, "did I wilfully and persistently do something of which he disapproved. He spoke to me about it when it was almost over, three or four words, in a low voice, nearly as an 'aside.' These words, the only unfriendly ones I ever had from him, remain deeply graven in my memory. However, when this episode was over, it was forgiven, if not forgotten, and it had no lasting influence on his attitude towards me. If I cannot now think of it without feeling a bit ashamed, this feeling is tempered by the thought: Only once in a lifetime, once in thirty-five years. That is not such a bad record."[34]

Sachs was not unaware of the narrow limits to which his independence had been pushed. It occurred to him to wonder, after Freud's death, whether he was more independent of Freud and less under his influence after his death than he was during his lifetime. The answer was that he neither thought so nor wished so. He reviewed the rules of thumb he had devised for his behaviour towards Freud soon after he became his disciple, and found that they still applied. His first rule had been to maintain a scientific attitude and accept nothing on authority, but to "try to be open-minded and take a favourable view of his opinions, however startling and astonishing they might seem at first sight." It was not due to his lack of free and unbiased judgment, he decided, "that in almost every case I became sooner or later fully convinced that he was right."

In practical matters Sachs considered it more advisable to spare Freud any friction than to protect himself against a *sacrificium intellectus*. If his opinion was opposed to Freud's, he did not hesitate to say so. Freud in his turn would always give Sachs full opportunity to express his point of view, and would listen willingly, but was rarely, if ever, influenced. "After that," Sachs recalled, "I acquiesced unreservedly with his decisions and acted in the way he wished."

In view of Sachs' abysmal self-abnegation, it is not surprising that Freud did not respect him. Sachs' excessive humility may have been his individual solution of how best to get along with Freud. But the demands which Freud made on his more submissive followers were likely to produce behaviour such as Sachs'. And once Freud had demanded and received this kind of unswerving deference, he abhorred it. That this was the case is shown by a personal letter he wrote at the time in which he described his followers as "this *crapule* which surrounds me."

There were other men among this group of early followers to whom Freud accorded a greater measure of respect. Significantly, these were the independent and ambitious men who would later break with him altogether rather than submit to the paternal ukase. These disciples best exemplified the self-reliance which Freud had won so dearly for himself. One was Otto Rank, brilliant, imaginative and unstable, who remained Freud's closest and most trusted collaborator for twenty years. He soon sat in the place of honour at Freud's left at the meetings of the Vienna Psychoanalytic Society. To him Freud delegated much of the responsibility of building up the psychoanalytic associations which began to be organized after 1908. Freud treated Rank as a favourite son. He had the highest appreciation for his energy, intelligence and originality. He did everything in his power to help and guide Rank and to smooth his path in life. He gave to him the most cherished gift in his possession—a leading part in the psychoanalytic movement.

In spite of the esteem and protection by which Freud had attempted to bind him, Rank broke away. It was a hard decision for him to make and he did it clumsily—alternately renouncing all his opinions, and then half-heartedly turning back to them. With the publication of his book tracing neurotic symptoms back to "the birth trauma"—a theory at variance with Freud's views—the rupture was complete. Freud would have no more truck with him. For the loss of a friend who had shared with him many of the traumatic birth pangs of psychoanalysis he showed no regret. He simply said: "*Wenn man jemanden alles verziehen hat, ist man fertig mit ihm.*" ("Now after I have forgiven everything, I am through with him.")

Alfred Adler was another early disciple whom Freud respected. The inevitable long, thin cigar clutched in his teeth, Adler from the start of the Wednesday evening meetings did not hesitate to hurl his own ideas at Freud. In his soft, slurred Viennese dialect, he would return again and again to his theory of the "inferiority of the organs." Himself a tiny man with the lust for power that seems to go so often with undersize, Adler believed that it was the feeling of weakness and inferiority, not sexual disorder, that was basic to neurosis. According to his ideas, the child wants to be a man, and the woman also, because the man is stronger than the woman or the child. In all weak creatures, Adler felt, this wish or will to power expresses itself in the same fashion. To this mechanism Adler had soon applied the tag of "masculine protest."

Even at the beginning of his association with Freud, Adler showed neither talent nor interest in the technique of psychoanalysis and the phenomena of the unconscious. He was, from the start, thoroughly dedicated to his Nietzschean *idée fixe* about the universal will to power. Freud, then as ever, was constitutionally incapable of absorbing ideas into the body of his theory which he had not himself first painfully developed in his own mind. So it was not Adler's idea which Freud respected. He appreciated instead the intensity of Adler's single-minded insistence on his idea; his courage in disputing the ideas of the master; and his ambition—those qualities which were so unmistakably the hallmarks of Freud's own character.

As he did with Rank, Freud singled Adler out, in those early years of psychoanalysis' development, for marks of special distinction. Adler too had his place of honour at the long table in the waiting-room. Later Freud had him appointed first head of the Viennese Psychoanalytic Society. But Adler was not to be deflected from his purpose. Wittels watched him at these early meetings and saw him prowling "as a cat prowls around a bowl of cream. A struggle was going on within him. It was not a struggle for knowledge, seeing that he had his ideas already finished in his mind. It was a struggle for the courage to bear testimony when he knew that this could not fail to lead to a breach between himself and Freud."[35]

But before Adler had summoned up sufficient courage to force the breach, a group of new disciples—outlanders—had been attracted to Freud's doctrines. Their allegiance was to begin to change the character of the nascent psychoanalytic movement from an auto-intoxicating Viennese ferment to a scientific mainstream of international proportions. They were not, however, to change the character of the father of the psychoanalytic movement. The character that was his "destiny" was to continue to produce the same effect on the newer disciples it had on the earlier ones. And this new growth, together with its inevitable aftermath of disruptions, was to strengthen in Freud his Messianic conviction that his and his alone was the Word and the Law.

9

See How It Splits

The first psychiatrists in the world to recognize and apply Freud's doctrines in public practice were Eugen Bleuler, director of the Burghoelzli Clinic of Psychiatry in Zürich, and his chief assistant, Dr. Carl Gustav Jung. While the growing awareness of psychoanalysis among psychiatrists at this time resulted everywhere in a violent repudiation of it, in Zürich the temperate Swiss were largely in agreement with Freud. As early as 1902 Jung had published a work on occult phenomena which contained a favourable reference to Freud's theory of dream interpretation. And by 1903 or 1904, Bleuler and Jung had begun to apply Freud's theories in treating the Burghoelzli patients. Shortly thereafter they urged the entire clinical staff to learn and test the Freudian method.

By 1907, when an aspiring psychiatrist, Abraham Brill, arrived at Burghoelzli to study, he found that the spirit of Freud permeated the entire hospital. Staff conversation at meal-time was liberally salted with such words as "complex" and "repression." No doctor was permitted to make a slip of any kind without the others demanding that he explain it according to Freud. Wives and female internees, unembarrassed by the flow of uninhibited talk, were just as eager to discover the concealed Freudian mechanisms as their husbands. The Burghoelzli also boasted a Psychoanalytic Circle which met monthly. Not all who attended agreed unequivocally with Freud's views. But the meetings on the whole were fruitful and promoted a wider understanding of Freud's theories.

Psychiatry, as Brill had known it before, had been devoid of interest and barren of hope: It had consisted of labelling and classifying the disorders the patient suffered from—this form of dementia præcox, or that kind of manic-depressive insanity. At the Burghoelzli, the infiltration of Freud's point of view had changed all that. There Brill found that "we focused our interest on the particular expressions of the patient. Instead of simply saying that the patient had hallucinations of hearing, we wished to know why he heard these particular voices; for, following Freud, we invariably found that these particular hallucinations could be perceived only by this particular patient. They told the struggles of his wrecked individual life."[36]

Many of the physicians who worked at the Burghoelzli at the time were later to play a large part in the history of the psychoanalytic movement—among them Riklin, Karl Abraham and Meier. Of all the staff, however, none was so ardent a Freudian as Jung. Able, enthusiastic, impulsive, he permitted no disagreement whatever with Freud's views. He grew intolerant and angry with anyone who ventured to doubt so much as a single psychoanalytic tenet. With his immediate grasp of what Freud was saying, and his intuitive recognition of the unconscious phenomena Freud had charted, he quickly became an extremely gifted interpreter of dreams and a psychoanalytic practitioner. As a teacher of the new doctrine, he was both impressive and vehement. At about this time he published his *Psychology of Dementia Præcox,* which started the younger European psychiatrists thinking and the older ones fuming, and which established him as a pioneer psychoanalyst in psychiatry. Although Director Bleuler had begun the psychoanalytic ferment in Zürich, it was Jung who emerged as its foremost Swiss champion.

Back in Vienna, Freud was delighted at the news of the work being done by Jung and the Burghoelzli. In no other city could he find such a devoted group of adherents, or a public clinic thrown wide open to psychoanalytic investigation; or, for that matter, a clinical teacher of great talent who considered psychoanalytic principles an integral part of the study of psychiatry. Only in Zürich at the time was there an opportunity to learn the new science and apply it in practice. And Freud began to think of Zürich as the site of the "infective lesion" which would spread the "psychic epidemic" of psychoanalysis.

He placed an inordinate amount of hope in these first foreign followers of his, just as he had in his first Viennese followers. Now at last, after a decade of landlock in Vienna, the doctrines he had dredged from the abysses of his own struggle with himself were beginning to be officially recognized beyond the borders of his native land. This recognition, stemming from the placid, protected Protestant valleys of Switzerland, constituted a soothing balm which he could apply to the wounds of humiliation inflicted by the Viennese psychiatrists. The Swiss were not tormented Jews, as the Viennese were. Instead, they belonged to the safe and sheltered world of Christianity. And Jung, tall, straight, clean-shaven and close-cropped, had the look of a young Siegfried.

Jung undoubtedly symbolized to Freud acceptance by the Aryan world. And Freud found in Jung a brother-in-arms, a soldier valiantly dedicated to the lonely crusade. No wonder, then, that Freud was shortly to express these feelings by designating Jung as his heir apparent.

The Swiss were by no means mere passive recipients of Freud's teaching—they were producing important original contributions of their own along psychoanalytic lines. Through their use of Wundt's association experiment, they were building a bridge between experimental psychology and psychoanalysis—getting quick laboratory confirmation of psychoanalytic facts.

More important than this, since experimental confirmation offered no essential contribution to the psychoanalytic technique, was the original work of Bleuler and Jung. Bleuler, in one of his books, pointed out that many psychotic phenomena could be interpreted by psychoanalytic procedure, just as dreams were. And a little later in 1911, in his book on schizophrenia, he accorded the psychoanalytic point of view equal stature with the older clinical one for an understanding of the disease. Jung had, in his *Psychology of Dementia Præcox,* applied the psychoanalytic method to an understanding of the most obscure phenomena of dementia præcox and had thereby made important findings about the origin of the disease. So conclusive was the evidence he presented that from that time on it became impossible for psychiatrists to ignore psychoanalysis.

Jung made a further contribution which the world soon seized on, but which Freud never regarded very highly. He spoke of "the complexes" in describing the groups of neurotic ideas and feelings clustering around the core of an emotional disturbance. The word soon became a convenient and indispensable term for summarizing psychological facts. No other term newly minted in the psychoanalytic laboratory gained either such widespread popularity or such misuse and misapplication.

Out of the international traffic in psychoanalytic ideas grew the first Psychoanalytic Congress—held in Salzburg in 1908. This was the first time that men of various countries met to discuss psychoanalytic affairs. True, the "world" at Salzburg was represented mainly by adherents from Zürich and Vienna, with a sparse spattering of devotees from London (Ernest Jones) and Budapest (Ferenczi). But a start was made towards a wider dissemination of psychoanalytic information: a periodical was organized and began to appear in 1909, under the jawbreaking name of *Jahrbuch fuer Psychoanalytische und Psychopathologische Forschungen,* edited by Bleuler and Freud with the help of Jung. The close tie between the schools of Vienna and Zürich found expression in this publication for the next few years.

Those propagandist measures had their effect. By 1911, Havelock Ellis, who never became an adherent of psychoanalysis but always regarded it with sympathy, could write: "Freud's psychoanalysis is now championed and carried out not only in Austria and Switzerland, but in the United States, in England, India, Canada and, I doubt not, in Australasia." A doctor from Chile put in his appearance at the second International Congress to praise the results of psychoanalytic therapy in obsessions and to speak in favour of the theory of infantile sexuality. An English neurologist in India informed Freud that he had been using psychoanalysis on his Mohammedan patients.

But it was in America that Freud's theories were accorded their most respectful hearing. The enthusiastic Dr. Brill had returned to America from Zürich in the spring of 1908, and in New York he started at once to proselytize for psychoanalysis. He, too, met with opposition, but not of the kind Freud had known. Although the opposition was strong, and though for some years Brill remained the only practising psychoanalyst in America,* he was listened to with interest. The academic world which had shunned Freud in Europe was far more friendly to him in America.

In 1909, Professor G. Stanley Hall, president of Clark University at Worcester, Massachusetts, invited both Freud and Jung to attend the university's twentieth anniversary celebration and to lecture to a conference of psychologists on the origin and development of psychoanalysis. Freud and Jung were delighted to accept. With them came Ferenczi from Budapest, and the three were joined in Worcester by Brill and Jones.

At Clark, a small but respected university, Freud found to his great astonishment that the faculty was not only familiar with his work, but had been lecturing about it to the students. America amazingly, for all its "prudery" in Freud's mind, could regard his work without prejudice and discuss it freely where Europe dismissed it as offensive.

Although Freud never relinquished his preconceived poor opinion of America, and his remarks about it continued to be uniformly derogatory, he returned to Vienna with increased self-respect. "As I stepped on to the platform at Worcester to deliver my 'Five Lectures upon Psychoanalysis'," he later recalled, "it seemed like the realization of some incredible day-dream: psychoanalysis was no longer a product of delusion—it had become a valuable part of reality."

* Ernest Jones, however, was practising in Toronto.

But the warmth of the academic reception did not serve to change his opinion of America. Fatigued and irritable because of a digestive disorder that plagued him during his week's stay in the United States, Freud recalled bitterly, twenty-five years after his visit, that the only expression of sympathy he had received from his hosts was a perfunctory "That's too bad." He found America immature and repressed, and he never admitted the possibility of its change, although he never revisited it. Late in life, he dismissed the whole country in a casual remark to a friend: "America is the most grandiose experiment the world has seen, but I am afraid it is not going to be a success."

His dreary impressions of the country were undoubtedly reinforced by a letter Jung wrote him from America a few years after their joint visit. In it Jung said that he had discovered that soft-pedalling the role of sexuality for Americans had helped him to awaken interest in psychoanalysis. Freud could not tolerate this concealment and blamed Americans for needing it. Later he blamed American women for the parlous state of America's sexuality. He told a visitor in 1934: "American women are an anti-cultural phenomenon. They have nothing but conceit to make up for their sense of uselessness. You have a real rule of women in America. You young men go to college with girls, fall in love and marry at an age when the girls are usually much more mature than the men. They lead the men around by the nose, make fools of them, and the result is a matriarchy. That is why marriage is so unsuccessful in America—that is why your divorce rate is so high. Your average American man approaches marriage without any experience at all. You wouldn't expect a person to step up to an orchestra and play first fiddle without some training, but the American man steps into marriage without the least experience for so complicated a business. In Europe, things are different. Men take the lead. That is as it should be."

Here the browbeaten American meekly inquired: "But don't you think that it would be best if both partners were equal?"

"That," Freud said, "is a practical impossibility. There

must be inequality, and the superiority of the man is the lesser of two evils." He did, however, find something good to say of American women: "She hasn't got the European woman's constant fear of seduction."[37]

Women, it seemed, were much on Freud's mind during his visit to America. With his stomach upset, he missed his wife's sympathetic ministrations. He joined Jung at breakfast in Worcester one morning only to remark bitterly: "I haven't been able to sleep since I came to America. I continue to dream of prostitutes."

"Well," Jung shrugged, "why don't you do something about it?"

"But," Freud replied, appalled at the suggestion, "I'm a married man."

What with his indigestion, his homesickness, and the American women who stood in no fear of seduction, Freud's jaundiced eye viewed even the men who respected him enough to afford him scientific hospitality with analytic coldness. G. Stanley Hall, Clark's president, who was esteemed as a psychologist and educator, and who had some years before Freud's visit introduced psychoanalysis into his courses, Freud found to have a touch of "the kingmaker." With James J. Putnam, the noted professor of neuropathology at Harvard, Freud established warm personal relations. For years before Freud's visit Putnam had spoken disparagingly of psychoanalysis, but after meeting Freud he threw the whole weight of his universally respected personality into a defense of its cultural value. Despite this and the fact that Freud found Putnam to be personally an "estimable" man, he disliked the "ethical bias" of Putnam's character. This bias, he remarked somewhat gratuitously, sprang from "a reaction against a predisposition to obsessional neurosis." And there was reason to regret, in Freud's mind, Putnam's "inclination to attach psychoanalysis to a particular philosophical system and to make it the servant of moral aims."

Of all the men Freud met in America, he spoke with undiluted respect of only one—William James, the philosopher. Freud never forgot a scene that once took place as the two men walked together. James stopped suddenly, handed Freud a bag he was carrying and asked him to walk on, saying that he would catch up with Freud as soon as he had got through an attack of angina pectoris which was just coming on. A year later James was dead of that disease. "I have always wished," Freud wrote later, "that I might be as fearless as he was in the face of approaching death."

By the spring of 1910, when Freud called together a second congress of psychoanalysts at Nuremberg, he had conceived a project whose repercussions have not yet died away. By this time Freud had persuaded himself that in Jung he had found the ideal temporal head of his new religion. If Jung would run the secular affairs of the church—take over the external organization and regulation of psychoanalysis—then he, Freud, could concern himself exclusively with that which was nearest to his heart, the formulation of the dogma. He would be free to conduct his theoretical investigations. The disciples close to Freud at the time saw this wish as clearly as if it had been expressed. Wittels described Freud's attitude towards Jung as being: "This is my beloved son, in whom I am well pleased." And Brill heard the younger, more irreverent disciples refer to Freud and Jung as "Allah and his prophet."

Before Freud sprang his sensation at the second Congress held at Nuremberg, the little group of Viennese psychoanalysts and *aficionados*, first in seniority but second in the eyes of the master, had eyed the Zürichers with nervous apprehension. The Viennese, largely Jews, thought they sensed an Aryan scorn of them in Jung. The Zürichers, tidy Swiss Protestants—Pastor Oskar Pfister among them—feared "the far-fetched interpretations" of the Viennese, by which they meant the Viennese emphasis on sexuality.

What Freud proposed through the medium of Ferenczi at the Nuremberg Congress was that an International Psychoanalytic Association be founded, whose centre would be Zürich and whose perpetual president would be Jung. This meant that Jung, not Freud, would have absolute power to appoint and supervise all psychoanalysts; that all scientific writings of the members of the association would be submitted to him for approval before publication; in short, that the entire responsibility for the future development of psychoanalysis as a profession would be entrusted to Jung.

The Viennese, who had suspected their decline in Freud's estimation, had not suspected their utter downfall. On the afternoon of this dark day, they met secretly in the Grand Hotel in Nuremberg. Adler and Wilhelm Stekel, in particular, who were the current Viennese favourites, were determined to resist Ferenczi's proposal. Freud was called both ruthless and simple-minded. There was angry talk of his "*coup de main.*" There was equally angry comparison of Jung's protected power with the power of the Pope.

Into this outraged group Freud walked unbidden and greatly excited. The unexpected opposition of his hitherto docile followers had infuriated him.

"Most of you," he said, "are *Jews* and therefore you are incompetent to win friends for the new teaching. Jews must be content with the modest rôle of preparing the ground. It is absolutely essential that I should form ties in the world of general science. I am getting on in years and am weary of being perpetually attacked. We are all in danger." Then, seizing his coat by the lapels, he said, "They won't leave me a coat to my back. This Swiss will save us—will save me and all of you as well."[38]

It was out in the open finally—the fear and horror of being Jewish; the conviction, or rather the knowledge long unexpressed, that the accident of his birth was the greatest deterrent to his career. Pride, made deep by a deep hurt, would never again permit him to reveal himself in this way. On the contrary, it had already led him, before the never-to-be-repeated aberration of this incident, to seek identification with the members of his own faith, and thus to stand united with the ranks of the "incompetent" and "perpetually attacked."

Long before this outburst, at the time of his father's death, when he had realized the emotional facts of his life, he had faced the fact of his ancestry. The decision he arrived at then he stated succinctly years later: "My parents were Jews," he said, "and I have remained a Jew myself." In the years immediately after his father's death and psychoanalysis' birth, two currents of feeling united in him to make him seek conventional inclusion in the ranks of the Jews: he had won his first insight into the dark reaches of human instinctual life, and he had seen much which sobered and even frightened him. Combined with this, the publication of his discoveries left him outlawed and shunned.

In his isolation, he told the members of the B'nai B'rith, a Jewish organization, many years later: "The longing arose in me for a circle of chosen, high-minded men who, regardless of the audacity of what I had done, would receive me with friendliness. Your society was pointed out to me as the place where such men were to be found. That you were Jews only suited me the more, for I myself was a Jew, and it always seemed to me not only shameful but downright senseless to deny it."[39]

Freud had joined the B'nai B'rith society of Vienna ten years before the scene in Nuremberg's Grand Hotel. He joined them then, as he told them many years later when he was celebrating his seventieth birthday, not out of faith or national pride. For, he said, he had always been an unbeliever, raised without particular regard for the strictures of orthodox Judaism, but not without regard for the ethical demands of that religion. "Nationalistic ardour" he had always tried to suppress in himself, for he thought it not only pernicious and unjust, but also too similar to the spirit which moved "the people among whom we Jews live." Why then was the attraction of Judaism and Jews "irresistible," as he told the B'nai B'rith it was? The answer he gave them was this: that Judaism for him was made up of "many dark emotional forces, all the more potent for being so hard to grasp in words, as well as the clear consciousness of an inner identity, the intimacy that comes from the same psychic structure."[39]

This clear consciousness of an inner identity with Jews had not, understandably enough, hindered Freud from regarding Jung as the saviour of the psychoanalytic movement, and from suggesting him as its president in perpetuity. He had told the Viennese in anger the real reason for his choice of Jung. After the noise of the battle died down, at a time when he could sum up the emotional effect of the incident with a quotation from Goethe: "Cut it short. On doomsday 'twon't be worth a farthing"—he had plenty of rational reasons to offer. For one thing, he felt that psychoanalysis' identification with Vienna was an obstacle to its growth. Zürich, becalmed in the centre of Europe, where a psychiatrist of renown had already opened the doors of his institution to the new science, would afford psychoanalysis a much more benign climate.

For another thing, he assumed that his person and his personality formed a second obstacle. He was, he said bitterly, "either compared to Darwin and Kepler or reviled as a paralytic." He therefore thought it wise not only to push the city of psychoanalysis' birth into the background, but its founder as well. Moreover, he was fifty-four—no longer young—and he was oppressed by the burden of guiding the growth of his science as well as developing it. Jung, with his conspicuous talents, the contributions he had already made to psychoanalysis, his independence and his energy, seemed the obvious choice to assume this authority. Such a secular authority was imperative in Freud's eyes. It was important because Freud rightly feared the abuses to which psychoanalysis could be put once it gained popularity.

"I felt," said Freud, "that there should be a place that could give the dictum: 'With all this nonsense, analysis has nothing to do; this is not psychoanalysis.' " An authority was needed not only for the job of policing the quacks and charlatans who would and did appear in due time, but for the job of centrally formulating rules for instruction in how psychoanalysis should be practised; in training physicians; and as a body for friendly intercourse and the mutual exchange of ideas.

As far as Jung was concerned, Freud in retrospect could admit that he had made a mistake. Jung was an unfortunate choice, Freud later said. He was not only incapable of tolerating another's authority, but he was unfit to be an authority himself. And his energies were devoted, said Freud, to the unscrupulous pursuit of his own interests. But Jung had seemed prepared, Freud continued somewhat wistfully, "to give up for my sake certain race prejudices which he had so far permitted himself to indulge." [Again Freud had been betrayed by his hopes. Twenty-five years after the scene at the Nuremberg Congress, Jung chose to remain and edit a German psychological periodical after the Jews on its staff had been expelled by the Nazis. In 1934, this magazine published an article by Jung in which, after accusing Freud and Adler of establishing negative psychologies because as Jews they could see only faults and not virtues, he said: "On the other hand, the Aryan unconscious contains tensions and creative germs and has to live up to the task of its future. . . . The Aryan unconscious has a higher potential than the Jewish, and this is the advantage and also the disadvantage of a young people close to the barbarian. The Jewish psychology cannot understand this and considered it nonsensical. I warned the world of this and was therefore called an anti-Semite. Freud is responsible for this. He and his Germanic followers could not understand the German psyche. Have they been taught a better lesson by the powerful National Socialism at which the whole world looks with astonishment—a movement which pervades a whole people and is manifest in every German individual?"]'

Despite Freud's firm conviction in Nuremberg that he was right and the Viennese wrong, the fight ended in compromise. Freud won his points: that Jung be elected president and that Zürich be the home centre of psychoanalysis. But the presidency was limited to a two-year term, and the centre of psychoanalysis was to be the home city of the president, changing with each election. Beyond this main issue, certain good had been accomplished: three local groups for the training of psychoanalysts and the uniform dissemination of analytic procedures had been established—one in Berlin under the administration of Karl Abraham, who had followed Freud loyally for a number of years; one in Zürich under the chairmanship of Jung; and one in Vienna, whose chairmanship, in a vain effort to appease Adler's wounded sensibilities, Freud had relinquished to Adler. A fourth group in Budapest, headed by Ferenczi, was formed later. (Bleuler had not attended the Congress because of ill health. Nor was he eager to join the new international association. Upon Freud's urging he did, however, join, only to resign shortly thereafter because of, as Freud says, "disagreements at Zürich." With Bleuler's resignation, the link between the Zürich group and the Brughoelzli hospital was broken.)

Notwithstanding the fact that the point at issue had been settled by compromise, bad blood was left on the Nuremberg battlefield. A three years' battle within the camp of the psychoanalysts had been joined—a battle that was to end in two great secessions. In Freud's mind, it was waged over an irreconcilable difference in scientific principles. In the minds of future minor defectionists like Wittels and Stekel, it was a struggle for power. "Three at least of the protagonists," said Wittels darkly, "—Freud, Jung and Adler—had the lust of domination."

Back in Vienna, it became increasingly apparent that Adler, despite his elevation to head of the Viennese group, chafed under his domination by Freud. This extremely ambitious little man, who seemed to have become imbued with a Messianic conviction only slightly less virulent than Freud's, felt that he was persecuted. He was brilliant, with a special gift for speculative thinking, but his gifts were soon overshadowed, in Freud's mind, by what he came to regard as Adler's "ungovernable mania for priority." Once, at a meeting of the Vienna Psychoanalytic Society, Adler claimed priority for the viewpoint of the dynamic conception of neurosis, a concept basic to and inherent in Freud's earliest work. At another time he asked the group, although the question was directed at Freud: "Do you believe that it is such a great pleasure for me to stand in your shadow my whole life?"

On the merits of his psychology, which by this time he had built into an airtight structure, Adler had no doubt whatever—just as Freud entertained no doubt that *he* was right. Of Adler's psychology, Freud was scornful—although he was later sufficiently impressed by Adler's exclusive emphasis on the psychology of the ego, or conscious self, to start paying added attention to it himself. Freud thought of Adler's psychology as a "system" in which all the corners had been dovetailed, the parts neatly glued together, and all consummated in a particularly arbitrary and artificial fashion. He himself, he thought, had been careful not to do this with psychoanalysis: he had painstakingly built up his theory on the foundation of clinical observation, and at the time he was keeping his theory in step with his clinical facts. Adler, he felt, had done the reverse—started out with a preconceived theory, "organic weakness," and fitted his facts into that. He was prepared to admit that Adler had made some important contributions to the psychology of the ego—"superfluous but admissible" he called them; but he felt that Adler had simply translated many of the facts of psychoanalysis into his own jargon, and that in doing so he had twisted and distorted those facts. The cardinal sin he found in Adler's structure was his denial of the importance of the unconscious and of the sexuality by which Freud set so much store. "Adler is so consistent in this," Freud said derisively, "that he considers the desire to dominate the woman, to be on the top, as the mainspring of the sexual act." And he went on to say, "The view of life which one obtains from Adler's system is founded entirely upon the impulse of aggression. It leaves no room at all for love. One might wonder that such a cheerless aspect of life should have received any notice whatever; but we must not forget that humanity, oppressed by its sexual needs, is prepared to accept anything if only the 'overcoming of sexuality' is held out as bait."[42]

With Adler and his adherents—by this time Adler had a score of followers who, like himself, were all Socialists—at sword's point with Freud, and with Freud as uncompromising in his views as Adler, the Wednesday evening meetings in the waiting-room lost their resemblance to a devotional. The opposing factions bitterly contested each other's claims, as one religious sect might the dogma of another. Before the meetings degenerated into an open brawl, Freud intervened. He said that his waiting-room was too small—for many new faces were now appearing at the meetings—and removed the group to the chill, uncongenial halls of the Viennese Medical Society.

Until the spring of 1911, Freud did his utmost to try to reconcile the opposing interests of the two groups. Not that he spared his opponents—he criticized them sharply, and his words often cut painfully. But he never descended to personalities and he tried to keep the furor on a plane of dispassionate scientific discussion. This was a vain effort. There was a constant transfer of allegiance from one camp to another, for among many of the embattled members personal antipathies were stronger than allegiance to doctrine. Two members, hating a third in common, would for a time be united by their common aversion—only to split apart again when a more consuming hate made itself apparent. Petty disputes gave way to whining remonstrances. Freud, who sat in the middle of the rivalry anxious only to be left in peace to work, grew as irritable as the father of an unruly brood. Polemics, jealousy, personal criticism, rival claims for priority, insults and wounded egos obscured the fire of comradeship which still burned pallidly.

In the spring of 1911 Freud, weary of the incessant wrangling, asked Adler once and for all to present a connected, prepared and orderly exposition of his ideas to the group. Three Wednesday evening meetings were allotted to his presentation. Only on the fourth evening, when Adler had entirely finished speaking his piece, was discussion permitted. Wittels, who was present and whose allegiance at the time belonged to Stekel, not to Freud, saw the scene through a red haze. The Freudian adherents, he said, "made a mass attack on Adler, an attack almost unexampled for its ferocity even in the fiercely contested field of psychoanalytic controversy. . . . Freud had a sheaf of notes before him and, with gloomy mien, seemed prepared to annihilate his adversary. . . . On the fifth evening a member proposed that Adler should be invited to leave the Society. . . . This was the not altogether creditable way in which Freud finally alienated the most notable among his disciples. Adler's resignation was accompanied by that of nine of his adherents."[43] Among these nine were men who did not wholeheartedly share Adler's views. Their decision had been influenced by Freud's high-handed tactics and their conviction that the whole procedure had violated the "freedom of science." As Sachs said: "It may well be that Freud's incisive and harsh criticism had hurt softer feelings and made them willing to think that Adler's complaint of intolerance was justified."

Wittels' animus and inaccuracy—Jung, not Adler, was at that time Freud's favourite—are evident. But his account of the session is valuable as an indication of the passion that was released when an irresistible force, Freud, met an immovable object, Adler. His account is evidence, too, of the passion that is engendered when the founder of a religion meets in the ranks of his own followers a rival prophet who is bent on promulgating another religion. Rather than incorporate Adler's ideas into the body of his own, Freud preferred that Adler leave the psychoanalytic fold altogether.

Adler and his splintered Adlerians had seceded or been excommunicated from the psychoanalytic church before the Third Congress was held at Weimar in 1911. By the time the Fourth Congress met at Munich in September, 1913, the psychoanalytic climate was overcast with another war cloud. While Freud had been engaged in the battle of Vienna, the Zürichers had also been arming for a war of independence. The first note of strife had been struck as far back as the Nuremberg Congress when one of the Swiss analysts had arisen to say that it was a mistake to lay so much stress upon sexuality. A year later, another member of the Zürich school had published some articles in which he asserted that psychoanalysis had fortunately begun to overcome some of its initial regrettable mistakes, and was thus emerging on to the high road of respectability. And in 1912 Jung had written his letter to Freud from America, in which he had told of winning friends by soft-pedalling the sexual factor in psychoanalysis. This piece of intelligence had infuriated Freud.

At the Munich congress the antagonisms between the Zürichers and the Viennese, which had been secretly growing for three years, burst into the open. The final straw was Jung's *Wandlungen und Symbole der Libido* which had appeared in print shortly before the congress convened. In it Jung asserted that dreams gave expression to the divine in man as well as to the animal. Freud, who considered any serious reference to man's divinity as so much twaddle, was considerably annoyed. On the floor of the congress he declared that the work and inferences of the Swiss could "not be regarded as legitimate developments of psychoanalysis." Jung, who was prepared to meet fire with fire, as chairman of the proceedings limited the time allowed to each man who presented a paper, and allowed unlimited discussion in the intervals. During discussion, the storm of invective, attack and riposte mounted. Just how Freud felt as his crown prince emerged as the leader of a fully-fledged palace revolt he never revealed directly. In his only published reference to the battle, Freud wrote in the style of the French newspaper which described a particularly brutal murderer as "*cet indélicat*," that Jung presided over the meeting in "an unamiable and incorrect fashion" and that the proceedings were "fatiguing and unedifying."

For all his attempt to dismiss the cleavage as unimportant, he suffered from a deep-seated conviction that he had been betrayed by the man in whom he had invested the most trust and hope. Twenty years after the event, a casual visitor was startled by Freud's bitterness about Jung, a bitterness which he said "was always apparent and extended from [Jung's] person to his countrymen." (This bitterness would also manifest itself in arrogance. Once, in speaking of the secessionists, Freud remarked: "Does one know today with whom Columbus sailed when he discovered America?") With the same visitor Freud discussed a dream of Jung's, which Jung had described to him six months before the break occurred. From this dream, said Freud—still concerned, although he had passed his seventy-fifth birthday—he should have known what was about to happen.

To another visitor of this same period, Freud revealed a curiously mixed residue of feeling for Jung without mentioning him by name: "Personal differences—jealousy or revenge or some other kind of animosity—always came first," he said, "scientific differences later. If people were really friendly, differences of scientific opinion would not make enemies of them. . . . It is people of talent who are responsible for these theories that are floating around and confusing the scientific world. It is not the stupid people who cause trouble. Stupid people ruin themselves—it is the people with talent who cause trouble. The reason for so much bad science is not that talent is rare—not at all. What is rare is character. People are not honest. They don't admit their ignorance and that is why they write such nonsense."[44]

The break with Jung* was undoubtedly one of the most instructive and painful lessons of Freud's life. To the job of demolishing both Jung and Adler as men and as scientists Freud brought all the power of his pen. He tired neither of finding new arguments to direct against them nor of urging his loyal followers to join the battle. But because his respect for Jung was greater than it was for Adler, his contemptuous dismissal of Jung's deviations from psychoanalysis was far more venomous than it was for Adler.

In Adler's psychology, despite Freud's dislike for it, he could find some good: it was consistent, coherent, and it was still founded on Freud's theory of the instincts. Of the two secessionist schools, Freud thought Adler's the more important. (The world has judged otherwise.) For Jung's modification of psychoanalysis, which substituted an emphasis on ethics and religion for sex, Freud had only adjectives like "unintelligible, muddled and confused." For Jung's refusal to see sexual maladjustment as the root cause of neurosis Freud had an analytic explanation: Jung's religious background held him as securely chained

* Despite the stormy proceedings at the Munich Congress, Jung was re-elected as president of the International Psychoanalytic Association for another two-year period. After this term was served the Freudians and the Jungians retired to their separate camps to vow undying hatred.

as Adler's Socialist record. This theme Freud embroidered in an unusual way: "I will encroach upon the realm of parables," he wrote in criticizing Jung, "and will assume that in a certain society there lived an upstart who boasted of descent from a very noble family not locally known. But it so happened that it was proved to him that his parents were living somewhere in the neighbourhood and were very simple people indeed. Only one way out remained to him and he seized upon it. He could no longer deny his parents, but he asserted that they were very aristocratic by origin, but were much reduced in circumstances, and secured for them at some obliging office a document showing their descent. It seems to me that the Swiss workers had been obliged to act in a similar manner. If ethics and religion could not be sexualized, but must be regarded as something 'higher' from the very beginning, and as their origin from the family and Œdipus complexes seemed undeniable, then there was only one way out: the complexes themselves could not from the beginning have had the significance which they seemed to express, but must have that higher . . . sense . . . which adapts them for proper use in the abstract streams of thought, of ethics and religious mysticism."[45]

As far as Freud could see, all the variations which Jung introduced into psychoanalysis originated from his desire to eliminate Freud's emphasis on sexuality. Jung's *Analytic Psychology* Freud called a "religio-ethical system." Therapy via this method Freud dismissed completely. He considered that Jung had substituted ethical encouragement and religious meditation for his own analytic technique.

For the public eye, Freud would bear the loss of Jung with equanimity. "Men are strong so long as they represent a strong idea," he wrote. "They become powerless when they oppose it. Psychoanalysis will be able to bear this loss and will gain new adherents for those lost. I can only conclude with the wish that fate may grant an easy ascension to those whose sojourn in the underworld of psychoanalysis has become uncomfortable. May it be vouchsafed to the others to bring to a happy conclusion their works in the depth."[46]

With his father's death Freud had learned a hard lesson—never again to seek a patron. With the excommunication of Jung from the psychoanalytic church, Freud learned another lesson—never again to seek an heir apparent. From this time on, he would work with many, depend on few, and never single out one man to inherit his mantle. He was fifty-seven when Jung departed the fold, and he was already committed by constant iteration to a path of "splendid isolation." The isolation would neither be so solitary nor so heroic as he continued to imagine it. But he was, despite the hosts of new followers and new admirers his work would win, despite his wife and six children, a man emotionally alone.

10

Husband and Two Fathers

Freud's emotional isolation was not new. Its seeds had been sown in his boyhood relationship with his family. And they had reached their first growth after his marriage to Martha Bernays when his work assumed so marked an ascendancy over his personal life that it became his real love. Early in their marriage he came to regard his wife with the same analytic detachment he regarded a neurotic symptom.

For this reason Freud's married life was extraordinary. Outwardly, the marriage was as orthodoxly correct as Freud's morals. Inwardly, as Freud unconsciously revealed, it lacked lustre and joy. It was as if Freud's capacity for love, naturally great, were encased in a block of ice.

That Freud's marriage was not based on a hasty and *grande passion* is evident. In the first place, it was never within the bounds of Freud's character to be swayed by passion. In the second place, he married Martha at thirty, after having kept her waiting for five years. Lastly, as he himself took pains to point out in his work, there is no such thing as psychic chance. We make mistakes, accidents happen to us, he said, because the unconscious has a will of its own which differs from our conscious will, and because the unconscious does what it pleases with us when our strictly logical attention lapses for a moment.

Thus, on the basis of Freud's own analysis of human motivation, a woman of Martha Bernays' type was what he unconsciously wanted: a woman who would not share in the intellectual life which became his consuming passion; a woman who would free him completely, by taking superb care of his physical needs, to pursue his own ends in his own way. A woman, in short, whose function resembled his mother's. To begin with, Freud had a circumscribed and Victorian view of women's rôle in life: he was convinced that women should submerge their identities and individualities in the services of their husbands and children. In Martha Bernays, who never for an instant dreamed of meeting her husband on an equal plane, he found just that.

She could not, however, give him what it was not in her power to give. After fifteen years of marriage, the limitations of her personality had begun to loom large in Freud's mind. In her domain of catering to his physical comfort and shielding him from the routine stresses of everyday living, she remained superlative. But she could not be as immediately sensitive to the other needs of his nature.

What Freud thought of his little Hamburg wife at times emerges clearly from his interpretation of his dreams. One of these dreams concerned a young woman patient whom he called Irma and an intimate woman friend of hers. These two reminded him of another young woman—a governess he had once treated. In the course of trying to discover what these three women meant in his ilfe and what the characteristics he attributed to them signified, he said: "Now only a few features remain which I can assign neither to Irma nor to her friend: pale, puffy, false teeth. The false teeth led me to the governess* . . . Here another person to whom these features may allude, occurs to me. She is not my patient, and I do not wish her to be my pa-

* This governess he had already described by saying that she "at first produced an impression of youthful beauty," but "upon opening her mouth took certain measures to conceal her dentures." It will be recalled that Martha Freud impressed people with her governess-like mien.

tient, for I have noticed that she is not at her ease with me, and I do not consider her a docile patient. She is generally pale and once when she had not felt particularly well, she was puffy." Here he breaks off as if he could not bear to uncover himself so nakedly. It is in a footnote that he reveals the identity of this other woman: "The complaint of pains in the abdomen" [which Irma, the girl in the dream, suffered from], he says, ". . . may also be referred to this third person. It is my own wife, of course, who is in question; the abdominal pains remind me of one of the occasions on which her shyness became evident to me. I must admit that I do not treat Irma and my wife very gallantly in this dream, but let it be said in my defense that I am measuring both of them against the ideal of the courageous and docile female patient."

Possibly this defense in Freud's mind was sufficient to acquit him of a lack of gallantry. It does not, however, acquit him of a more serious indictment: a merciless lack of charity towards his wife, which the dream records. "I have noticed," he said, "that she is not at her ease with me." He will not permit her to enter the sacred domain of his work—"I do not wish her to be my patient." Thus, with a stroke of the pen, he dismisses his devoted servant who, it appears, irks him for a failure to live up to the "ideal" proportions of that quality which so surely characterizes her.

Thus Freud pictures the woman who served him faithfully for more than a half-century: Martha was "pale, puffy," the wearer of false teeth; ailing, shy, timid, docile to a fault—yet not docile enough. Surely a unique description in the records of marriage relationships! She is not endowed in his dream thoughts with a single redeeming grace. And what more revealing comment is there to make about the wife of this husband than that she did not feel at ease with him?

It is true that had other husbands obeyed so unflinchingly the demands of pure science and compelled themselves to disclose their most secret feelings, Freud would not have emerged in the naked fashion he does as the unabashed exemplar of marital disenchantment. In the course of interpreting his dreams he says as much: "It cannot be denied that great self-control is needed to interpret one's dreams and to report them. One has to reveal oneself as the sole villain among all the noble souls with whom one shares the breath of life."

It is also true that this dream with its bitter associations may have been the reflection of a passing mood—that Freud might have felt particularly provoked with his wife at the time. But even if it were, the fact would nevertheless remain: a marriage built not on the mutual respect of two equals, but on the limitless subservience of the woman to the man is likely to generate just that uneasiness in the wife and irritation in the husband which Freud so faithfully recorded. Moreover, Freud made it quite plain that he did not consider his wife a fit guardian for their children in the event of his death. He wrote: " . . . a member of my household of whom I hope—for she is younger than I—that she will watch over the future of my children." This is undoubtedly an allusion to Minna, his wife's sister, who because of her independence and intellectual stature was always more companionable to Freud than his wife. But one guardian is not sufficient to make up for what he must have come to regard as his wife's unfitness. "My friend Otto," he says in a subsequent passage of his confession, "is the person whom I have asked to take charge of the physical education of my children—especially during the age of puberty—in case anything should happen to me."

For his recognition of the deep-rooted division between himself and his wife, Freud would sometimes reproach himself. He dreamed once of a monograph on the cyclamen which made him recall that this was Martha's favourite flower. And he says, "I reproach myself for remembering so seldom to bring her flowers, as she would like me to do." He recalls that the artichoke might be called his favourite flower, and says, "My wife, more thoughtful than I, often brings this favourite flower of mine home from the market." And he is reminded by other images in the dream of an old reproach often directed against him by his friends and family—that he is "much too absorbed in his hobbies."

On one occasion he forgot to call for his wife on time at a theatre she had attended alone. After mentioning this lapse, he delivered himself of the following: "Duties towards women (like army service) demand that nothing related to them must be subject to forgetting, and thus imply that forgetting may be permissible in unimportant matters but in weighty matters, its occurrence is an indication that one wishes to treat them as unimportant: that is, that their importance is disputed." This judgment reminds him inevitably enough of another conqueror of unexplored regions linked to a woman of lesser stature.

For his children, two of whom were now old enough to fight in the approaching war, Freud felt a deeper concern. For he could regard them as extensions of his own personality. The three boys—Martin, Oliver and Ernst—and the three girls—Mathilde, Sophie and Anna—had been named not according to the fashion of the day, but, on Papa's insistence, for people dear to his memory. Martin had been named "Jean-Martin" after Charcot. Anna had been named after Freud's sister. As Freud said, "The children's names make them *revenants*." In other words, they linked his past to his future.

Regarding them, then, as he did—primarily as instruments of destiny and immortality*—he came eventually to eye them with the same clinical dispassion he applied to everything in his life. It was not that he was not enormously fond of them. He was. But the warmth that smouldered within him was so carefully banked by considerations of "ought" and "should," and by the pattern of his relationship to his own father, that it rarely found expression in a spontaneous flow of affection.

Most of Freud's friends and co-workers were impressed by his great love for all children and by his charming naturalness and amiability with them. He could on occasion throw off the preoccupations of his day for a romp

* H. D., the poetess, once said that when Freud spoke of his children, "it was so tribal, so conveniently Mosaic. . . . It seemed the eternal life he visualized was in the old Judaic tradition. He would live forever like Abraham, Isaac and Jacob in his children's children, multiplied like the sands of the sea."[47]

with his children. After work, he would ascend the stairs to the family quarters, usually announcing his arrival with a sound between a grunt and a growl manufactured for the amusement of his youngest and favourite child, Anna. But these interludes of playfulness were rare. On the whole, the fact that he kept the natural depth of his feeling for them walled in more than offset the advantages of his great theoretical knowledge about the nature of childhood. Like his father, he expected his children to look up to him reverently. Like the filial injunctions implicitly laid down by his father, Freud expected his children to honour and obey him unquestioningly. The atmosphere of rigid Jewish ethics which he fought so furiously he succeeded in recreating in his own household. Just as the sons of his spirit in psychoanalytic circles were expected to accept his dictates without exception, so his own children were expected to accede to his authority. At home, as abroad, his word was the law.

It was not only his wife who revolved around the sun that was "der Papa." The children were also expected to fit their expanding lives into the prescribed pattern his life demanded. Friends of the family often joked about the awed way in which the children referred to everything pertaining to their father. A story made the rounds of his disciples: When one of the children had been away from the house for a time and was met by another, it was said, the child who had been at home was quick to pass on the latest development in the household: "Father now drinks his tea," the story made the child say, "from the green cup instead of from the blue one." As the children grew, their awe for him grew. But it grew neither as fast nor as luxuriantly as his own patriarchal, Mosaic attitude towards them.

Instead of the spontaneous simple affection, which it was not in Freud's nature to give his children, he wore for them the same air of sceptical inquiry with which he had equipped himself to face the world.

He tells us: "One of my boys, whose vivacious temperament was wont to put difficulties in the management of nursing him in his illness, had a fit of anger one morning because he was ordered to remain in bed during the forenoon, and threatened to kill himself. . . . In the evening, he showed me a swelling on the side of his chest which was the result of bumping against the door knob. To my ironical question why he did it, and what he meant by it, the eleven-year-old child explained, 'That was my attempt at suicide which I threatened this morning.' "[48] He wrote, early in the century: "When a member of my family complains that he or she has bitten his tongue, bruised her finger and so on, instead of the expected sympathy, I put the question 'Why did you do that?' " But—as if in recognition that sympathy would be more natural in such circumstances—he followed this admission with: "But I have most painfully squeezed my thumb after a youthful patient acquainted me during the treatment with his intention . . . of marrying my eldest daughter while I knew that she was then in a private hospital in extreme danger of losing her life."[49]

However, under his attitude of ironical detachment from these episodes in the lives of his children, and apparently undetected by his children, there pulsed an archaic paternal love. When Mathilda, his eldest daughter, lay in danger of losing her life, Freud paced through a room in his bathrobe and straw slippers. His eye lit upon a beautiful little marble Venus, one of the treasures of his small collection, resting on a bracket attached to the wall. Suddenly, impulsively, he tore a slipper from his foot, hurled it at the Venus, and as it fell and broke into pieces, he recited in all calmness a verse from a German poet:

Ach! Die Venus ist perdu
*Klickeradoms!—von Medici!**

This "crazy action" and his calmness at the sight of the damage he explained thus: That morning he had heard that there had been a significant improvement in Mathilda's condition. He had said to himself: "After all, she will live." And within himself he must have decided that

* "Alas The Venus of Medici is lost!"

such good fortune deserved an act of sacrifice. "That I chose the Venus of Medici as this sacrifice," he said, "was only gallant homage to the convalescent." And in bafflement at his uncharacteristic fit of destruction he mused: "But even today it is still incomprehensible to me that I decided so quickly, aimed so accurately and struck no other object in close proximity."[50]

From the face Freud turned to them, the children could hardly have learned that their father loved them so violently. His love might burst out in acts of primitive sacrifice, but in their presence he was the restrained, contained Papa, an awesome, increasingly famous man. Because he never allowed himself fully to express his love for the children, the dammed-up emotion flowed out not only in the violence of sacrifice, but in the violence of over-concern, over-protection and over-anxiety. Freud worried constantly and unceasingly about his children's futures, and their fates, as individuals and, understandably, as Jews. This worry was so pervasive that he could not stop himself from discussing it with his patients and casual visitors. When he was still in his forties and in good health, and his children were hardly past their infancy, he had already been greatly concerned over who would care for them in the event of his death. As they grew older, his worry centred on what would happen to them as Jews.

As he had decided for himself at the turn of the century that he would remain a Jew, so he had decided for his children. At a time when Max Graf doubted the wisdom of raising his infant son as a Jew, for the child had been born in the midst of an anti-Semitic ferment whipped up by a Viennese demagogue, Freud said to him: "If you do not let your son grow up as a Jew, you will deprive him of those sources of energy which cannot be replaced by anything else. He will have to struggle as a Jew and you ought to develop in him all the energy he will need for the struggle. Do not deprive him of that advantage."[51]

Thus Freud's children were raised as Jews. They were raised as Jews at the same time as their father published article after book after monograph enlarging upon and documenting his thesis that at best all religion is an illu-

sion, at worst a universally practiced form of obsessional neurosis. They were not, of course, reared according to the letter of the religion of Freud's father. There was no observance of ritual—no Friday night candles, no attendance at synagogues, no taboos on food; but there was handed down to them the belief that as Jews they were to seek their identity with their co-religionists, as their father had decided to do. Thus Freud's children inherited from him the hard-won emotional attitude he had evolved towards the practical problem of his own religion, as distinct from his theoretical attitude towards religion as a whole.

Freud's concern over the fate of his children as Jews amounted almost to an obsession. This was so not only because of his own bitter history of isolation and discrimination, but because of the divergence between his scientific rejection of religion and his personal and familial acceptance of it. Because he continued to war with himself over the question of his religion, despite his apparent resolution of the problem, in his dreams the fate of his children constantly springs up from the dark chamber of his unconscious mind.

He wants them, these dreams say, to turn their handicap to advantage as he has done, and yet, like any father with any children, he wants to shield them from hurt. He suspects the secret content of their resignation to Judaism, as he knows the secret content of his own. For this reason it becomes clear that he feels that he and he alone—as if none of the children was capable of self-determination—can control the evil fate that leaned over their cradles and whispered: "You are Jews. You shall suffer as Jews." He says that the core of meaning of one of his dreams is the fear that "I shall have to leave my children to reach the goal of their difficult journey without my help." The children, he is convinced, cannot be trusted any more than he could trust himself, with the dignity of working out their personal solutions to salvation. They must, in a sense, atone for his own emotional sin of hating his father, and remain subservient to *his* will for them and his control.

Although by the time Freud broke with Jung his doctrines were already becoming instrumental in revolutionizing methods of child-rearing and in ushering in a new era of restriction-free *laisser-faireism* in education, he himself could not permit his children the privilege of self-determination. He could and did in small ways: he would, for example, admonish his children not to put on their company manners for guests. But the spirit of sporadic liberal exhortations like these was betrayed by the atmosphere of patriarchal authority which he generated. Papa's way of doing things was the right and only way for things to be done. Papa's dictates had to be carried out. Papa was a man of such unmistakable, albeit understated power, that no matter which way the children turned, they could not avoid the giant shadow he created. The only one of his children who would make a name for herself was the one who made no attempt to escape at all.

Freud, nearing sixty, had come a long way from the boyhood whose emotional boundaries had been set by his attempt to escape from his own father's arbitrary authority. He had come a long way, but he had travelled on the road marked "inevitable destiny." Thus, as a father to his own children, he had completed a full circle and arrived at a point remarkably similar to the one he had started out from. If he did not believe that his children "would never amount to anything" he would certainly never allow them the opportunity to find out for themselves.

Freud could not allow his spiritual sons in psychoanalysis any greater degree of self-determination or freedom than he could the children of his flesh. With Jung gone, and with him all hope of transferring to a trusted lieutenant the responsibility for the secular development of psychoanalysis, Freud had no choice but to assume the responsibility himself. He felt, justifiably enough in the face of the dangers from within and without in psychoanalysis, that it was just as vital for the new science to grow *sous cloche* under the protection of an international organization, as it was for it to develop clinically and theoretically.

Surrounded only by the loyal disciples—the "crapule"—Freud took on the job of temporal as well as spiritual head of the new science. He had to keep his brood in order. He had to see to it that uniform standards were established and rules formulated for the teaching and training of psychoanalysts and for their supervision. He had to stamp out intramural as well as extramural heresy. He had to make it clear who was entitled to describe himself as a psychoanalyst and who was not.

This was a heavy burden for a man of fifty-eight whose dearest wish was to be left free to pursue his scientific work in peace. At the time of the first World War his work had reached monumental proportions. Certain great truths, despite the heavy artillery and light cannon which had been brought to bear against psychoanalysis, and despite the impossibility of proof palatable to all corners, had emerged and were becoming widely accepted. Perhaps the greatest contribution of this first period of his work was the discovery of the dynamic and determining power of the unconscious mind. The fact that the unconscious is a part of our biological heritage as human beings; that it functions as consistently as the beat of our hearts or the reflexes of our muscles; and that it is as little amenable to our rational control as these organs—Freud established for all time. And in discovering the power of the unconscious mind over our conscious lives, Freud ended the dominance of the era of physiological psychology, and ushered in a new period whose concern was with the scientific understanding of man's inner life. This new psychological era was soon to permeate the thinking, the culture and the art of our time.

Other widely accepted Freudian truths had emerged by the beginning of World War I: the fact that dreams are meaningful and unfailing indicators of the state of this unconscious mind; the fact that psychoanalysis as a therapy had opened the way for the first time to a hopeful treatment of psychogenic disorders; the fact that the techniques of psychoanalysis cast a new and revolutionary light on the whole field of "normal" psychology and even on the study of organic disease. Controversy was almost stilled on certain of the basic terms and theories of psychoanalysis: the theories of repression and resistance and other forms of defenses of the ego, such as reaction-formation, projection and rationalization. Although

Freud's concept of the Œdipus complex continued to shock and be rejected by many, it would in a matter of a few decades become established as a lighthouse on the sea of man's emotional life. Soon there would be few left to quarrel with Freud's basic assumption that psychological functioning could be weighed, measured, observed and understood, just as physical functioning could be; and that this functioning followed specific laws, was never accidental, but always determined. In short, Freud had contributed in psychoanalysis a new scientific method, a new viewpoint and a new tool for the evolution of man as an emotional being.

But controversy would continue to rage over specific discoveries within the broad area of this acceptance, and eventually perhaps some of these specific theories would be rejected. Out of his discovery of the dynamics of the unconscious came Freud's postulates about mankind's instincts—a body of theory under current attack by a school of psychoanalysis which believes that man is more disturbed by his environment than by his inherited instincts. For Freud an instinct was not only an innate, automatically acting impulse, but any accumulation of energy in an individual which strove to express itself or to find an outlet. Instinctual energy was psychological energy. It could be compared with a fire. "If the fire rages uncontrolled in a house, we call it a disastrous conflagration; if it burns in a smelting furnace, we call it a useful industrial force. In other words, drives and impulses as they live within us are neither good nor bad, right nor wrong."[52]

Every organ of the body may be used by these impulses, Freud pointed out. As the energy accumulates in specific areas of the body, organs become tense. When tension increases sufficiently, the energy must break through as appetite, any appetite—the desire to eat, to scratch, to drink, to have sexual intercourse. In the moment of giving vent to this appetite or desire, pleasure is experienced. It was this process that Freud had studied in detail, and it was this process which he considered to be characteristic of all life forces. It was in naming the pleasure inherent in the process that Freud fell into a semantic trap; he called it "libidinous" or "erotic" or "sexual."

Because these words had until that time been exclusively associated with genital pleasure, Freud's theory of the instincts was immediately misunderstood and immediately labelled absurd. Freud had the intense man's need to express himself intensely. For this reason, some of the names and terms he used to describe psychological phenomena seem to some too metaphorical and too melodramatic. Freud's labelling of the "Œdipus complex," for example, connoting actual parricide, was unfortunate. Had he called the whole phenomenon by another name, it would undoubtedly have been recognized much earlier. What Freud was describing as "libidinous" and "erotic" were all the outcomes of the physiological processes characteristic of all organs of the human body, not the genital organs alone. Eating, drinking, exercising, artistic creation, inasmuch as they satisfied basic appetites, were all pleasure-seeking and pleasurable, thus hedonistic, and thus erotic. Or—to be more exact—this would be the outcome of the operation of all our instincts, if inhibition and repression, those willing handmaidens of civilization, had not been pressed into such universal service.

It is possible that Freud was led into giving a sexual name to a process which he did not conceive of as sexual in the usual sense, because of the depth and extent of the sublimation of his own sexual drive into creative work. It is true that, like the stock fictional character of the old maid who searches nightly under her bed in the hope of finding a robber, Freud tended to see sex where no sex ought to be. In any case, his thinking and writing about "libido" and sexuality underwent many changes and often appear to be contradictory or needlessly confused.

"I gave the name of libido to the energy of the sexual instincts and to that form of energy alone," Freud wrote. On the basis of this statement alone, Freud's chart of the underworld of man's emotional life might well be dismissed as "pan-sexual." But Freud's definition of sexuality differed from the traditional one. Freud saw sexuality as "divorced from its too close connection with the genitals, and . . . as a more comprehensive bodily function, having pleasure as its goal and only secondarily coming to serve the ends of reproduction. In the second place, the sexual impulses are regarded as including all of those merely affectionate and friendly impulses to which usage applies the exceedingly ambiguous word 'love.' I do not, however, consider that these extensions are innovations, but rather restorations; they signify the removal of inexpedient limitations of the concept into which we had allowed ourselves to be led."[53]

It was thus Eros or "love" in its original limitless sense as positive, creative, productive mover of the universe, not sex in its genital sense, that Freud saw as the core of man's instinctual life.

Most of that part of the scientific world of 1914-18 which was sufficiently interested in what Freud was saying to read him insisted, understandably enough, in view of his confusion of terms, on misunderstanding him. He added to the confusion by treating his postulate of the libido like so many ergs or kilowatts. Trained in the materialistic methods of Bruecke and Fechner, he described the development of his universal instinct towards all kinds of pleasure in a terminology devised for the description of physical phenomena. The libido was originally "non-centralized," he said. It might become "fixated" at various points of its development. If it is repressed, it "flows back" to its original point of fixation, and it is from this archaic vantage-point that "the energy breaks through" in the form of a symptom. Later on, it became clear to him that "the localization of the point of fixation" is what determines the choice of neurosis. Thus, because Freud remained wedded to an outworn scientific tradition fostered by the laboratories in which he received his training, he cloaked the formulation of a universal truth in garments unfashionable to the modern eye. In his zeal to fit his own original genius into the tradition he had been trained in, he allowed himself to be carried away. Some of the mechanistic descriptions of a phenomenon which had always belonged to the realms of philosophy or religion read as archaically to-day as some of the geographical descriptions of the pre-Columbus cartographers.

Much of what Freud charted within the realm of sexuality is now regarded as antiquated—like his concept that individuals may become fixated at immature levels of development where they are dominated by the pleasure they derive from their mouths or bottoms. For these "oral-" or "anal-sadistic" characters, Freud traced a whole series of respective characteristics. Indeed, he believed that their characters were formed completely by the failure of their libidos to reach a mature or genital stage of development. (But here again the conclusion that he reached would not have appeared half so absurd if his critics had not insisted on understanding these terms as either derogatory references to abnormal trends or fixation on the organs named. What Freud meant in typing people as "oral-" or "anal-sadistic" was that they had reverted for their pleasure to the satisfaction derived from original sources of instinctual energy—a conclusion neither so absurd nor naïve as many modern critics make out.)

Many of the conclusions Freud drew from his study of sexuality remain valid and valuable. He may have seen the love instinct myopically through the spectacles of a more naïve era, but he was none the less the first to attempt to dissect it within the scientific tradition of our time. And its development, as he traced it in broad outline, has become almost as widely recognized as the fact of our biological evolution from the ape. The sexual instinct, Freud found, contrary to the belief of his era, was operative from infancy, although at first it could not be discerned as such and did not operate independently of other instincts like hunger. It manifested itself at first through the activity of a number of related instincts—and these are all dependent upon "erotogenic" zones of the body. For the most part, this early sexual instinct found its object within the individual's own body. For this reason Freud termed this phase of development "auto-erotic." Later, the pleasurable gratifications derived from all parts of the body began to be centralized: first, in the nursing stage, in the pleasure derived from the mouth. This Freud termed the "oral" stage of libido development; second, in the gratifications derived from evacuation, in what he called the "anal-sadistic" stage. Only after the third and last stage has been reached does the primacy of the genitals establish itself and the sexual function begin to serve the goal of reproduction.

As the libido develops, it seeks an object for its affections. The first love-object, in the case of children of both sexes after they cease to find all their pleasure in their own bodies, is an incestuous choice—the mother. Later, but still in the first years of infancy, Freud says, the Œdipus complex becomes established; boys concentrate their sexual wishes upon their mothers, and, considering their fathers to be rivals, develop hostile impulses against them. Girls go through the same procedure, with the parents reversed.

The sexual life of man, he said, comes on in two waves, with an interlude of latency between them. Sexual concern and curiosity reach their first maximum growth between a child's fourth and fifth year. During this time, the male child is aware of his genitals, while the female child is confused about hers. The child does not think of the sexes as male or female but as "possessing a penis" or—in Freud's term—"castrated." From these observations Freud deduced the theory of the "castration complex" for the male, and "penis-envy" for the female, both of which he thought were profoundly important in the formation of character and neurosis. After the first sexual growth is nipped on the vine by repression, it is replaced by the latency period which lasts until puberty, and during which, said Freud, "the reaction-formations of morality, shame and disgust are built up." With puberty, the child's sexuality is reanimated, and with it the emotions clinging to his earliest love object and to his Œdipus complex. The sexual life of puberty, he said, "is a struggle between the impulses of early years and the inhibitions of the latency period."

That, in very broad and simple terms, is the way Freud traced the development of man's sexual function. He felt his assumptions to be no less true of normal people than of neurotics, children and perverts. "Looked at from the psychoanalytic standpoint," he said, "even the most eccentric and repellent perversions are explicable as manifestations of component instincts of sexuality which have freed themselves from the primacy of the genitals and are going in pursuit of pleasure on their own account, as they did in the very early days of the libido's development."[54] He had thus used his study of the sex life of neurotics as a jumping-off point for conclusions about the sex life of people in general. And he broadened the traditional concept of sexuality in another way: affection, friendly impulses, he said, were originally of a completely sexual nature, but had become inhibited in their aim or sublimated. "The manner in which the sexual instincts can thus be influenced and diverted enables them to be employed for cultural activities of every kind, to which indeed they bring the most important contributions."

His concern with sexuality led him into the formulation of ever new concepts and theories which have been almost universally criticized. The Œdipus complex in particular represented for him the trunk of a tree from which all kinds of flowering branches could be made to grow. Early in his clinical career, when Freud had successfully completed an analysis, he used to show the departing patient, in a kind of graduation ceremonial, a print of a picture by Ingres—"Œdipus Solves the Riddle of the Sphinx." His critics found his emphasis on Œdipus completely ludicrous. Individual psychoanalyses in the early days lasted a long time, as they do to-day. And in the first decade of the century they all led to the same conclusion. Amused at the monotony of the solutions, critics were fond of posing the question: "Wouldn't it be better to make it plain at the first consultation that the patient has committed incest with his mother and tried to poison his father?" None of this ridicule could deflect Freud from the conviction, based on his clinical experience, that the Œdipus complex was the nucleus of the neurosis. It was, he felt, not only the climax of the sexual life of a child, but it was the point of departure from which all later sexual development stemmed. But if this was the case, he reasoned, then the complex was no more native to a neurosis than it was to normal development. It must be true, he mused, "as Jung expressed it so well in the early days when he was still a psychoanalyst, that neurotics break down at the same difficulties that are successfully overcome by normal people."

With this discovery, Freud was more than content. It harmonized with his conviction that the depth psychology uncovered by psychoanalysis was in reality the psychology of the normal person. "Our path had been like that of chemistry," he concluded; "the great qualitative differences between substances were traced back to quantitative variations in the proportions in which the same elements were combined."

His feeling that the Œdipus legend was rooted not in fancy but in universal truth led him to penetrate further the structure of the normal personality. He came up first, in his effort to understand the objects with which the sexual drive sought to satisfy itself, with the theory of narcissism. Before the libido had become attached to the image of the parents, there was the earliest, auto-erotic stage of its development. In this state, Freud decided, the child's libido filled his own ego and had that for its object; the state could thereafter be called self-love, or narcissism. (The legendary Narcissus, the son of the Athenian river-god, had rejected the love of Echo, and fallen in love with his own image reflected in the water.) Reflection showed Freud that this narcissistic state never evaporated completely. All through an individual's life, he decided, "his ego remains the great reservoir of his libido, from which the attachment to objects . . . radiates out and into which the libido can stream back again from the objects. Thus, narcissistic libido is constantly being converted into object libido and vice versa."

The concept of narcissism represented the first time Freud had paid much attention to the mechanisms of the ego, or conscious self—a turn in his thinking possibly set off by the emphasis Adler had placed on describing the ego. Now, with the dualism that exerted so profound an influence on his own nature, he began to see narcissistic libido as a force opposed to the attachment of the libido to an outside object. The interests of self-preservation, he decided, which were imbedded in narcissism, defended themselves against the demands of object love. Early in the development of his libido theory, he had contrasted the libidinal instincts with such conflicting ego instincts as hunger and self-preservation. Now, with his recognition of narcissism, he posited a new dualism: the strife between narcissistic and object libido. Intentionally, this concept was kept somewhat vague, for Freud was not completely satisfied with it. The war years would replace it with a new and final dualistic concept of the eternal warfare staged by man's instincts.

The World War marked a rough dividing line in the course and tenor of Freud's work. Before 1914, he was primarily concerned with drawing conclusions from his clinical observations. After the war, although he never ceased to function as a great observer, his principal preoccupation became the formulation of psychoanalytic theory and the application of this theory to the interpretation of society as a whole. To the first period of his life's work belong some of his finest books, which have influenced the thinking of an era: *The Interpretations of Dreams* in 1900; *The Psychopathology of Everyday Life* in 1904; in 1905 two great works, *Wit and Its Relation to the Unconscious*, and *Three Contributions to the Theory of Sexuality;* and in 1913, the year of Freud's break with Jung, appeared the first and to most the finest of his investigations of religion, *Totem and Taboo;* a work which Freud called "an attempt to apply the results of psychoanalysis to unexplained problems of racial psychology," and which Thomas Mann called "a piece of world literature . . . a literary masterpiece allied to and comparable with the greatest examples of literary essays."

Besides these major works, there appeared between 1893 and 1917 a steady stream of invaluable monographs and articles on clinical problems—some sixty or seventy exclusive of the books. These papers ranged over a wide variety of subjects, but very generally they were all concerned with the formulation of what Freud had observed of the operation of the mutinous instincts that drive mankind. Some of the better known ones include: *Character and Anal Erotism* in 1908, which constituted Freud's first and, to many people, most disturbing contribution to the study of characterology; a study of the types of love life published in 1910; the formulation of the concept of anal-sadism in 1913; and in 1915, an important general study of character types.

In addition to these, there appeared works which presaged the turn Freud's thinking was to take during the war years. In 1907, a book of his called *Delusion and Dream in Jensen's "Gravida"* analyzed the relation of the unconscious, inner life of the artist to his artistic creation. In 1910 he published his second investigation of the unconscious life of the artist—a brilliant and imaginative study called *Leonardo da Vinci, a Study in Psychosexuality*. In 1914 there appeared a paper linked in theme to the analysis of religion in *Totem and Taboo*, but written out of a more directly personal need—*The Moses of Michelangelo*. This was the only paper Freud ever wrote which he felt called for anonymous publication. And in 1917, at a low ebb in his life, he looked back nostalgically to a happier era, and wrote a paper analysing certain childhood memories of one of his boyhood heroes—Goethe.

In general outline, this is what Freud accomplished in the first half of his life. Most modern psychiatrists recognize either explicitly or implicitly the fact that the greater part of Freud's clinical observations have been corroborated and have withstood the test of time. His theoretical contributions are another story. There the controversy rages unchecked. However, it is not within the province of this book to attempt to evaluate and judge Freud's work *per se*, but only in so far as it sheds light on the man himself and on the influence he has come to have.

There were, in the days of psychoanalysis' infancy during World War I, and there are now, in the days of its adolescence, numbers of critics who bridle at the amount of emphasis Freud placed on mankind's sexuality in general. There are psychoanalysts and informed laymen who think that Freud's libido theory is antiquated and somewhat absurd. There is a modern school of psychoanalysis which asserts that Freud is the victim of biological mechanism, Victorian myopia and assorted limitations which make his instinct theories archaic. There are critics who maintain that his classification of character into oral, anal and genital types is so much nonsense. The list of points of attack on this first period of Freud's work could be expanded indefinitely. Since, however, the ultimate proof of the psychoanalytic pudding is in the confessional, since its evidence is of necessity neither statistical nor experimental, but empirical, the question of upon whose side the God of truth is really enlisted must necessarily remain moot.

Freud disliked the arena to which the secular, international affairs of psychoanalysis led him. He was attacked by the outside world, but he was also attacked intramurally. Jung and Adler had departed, trailing the odour of battle. Minor satellites like Stekel, Wittels, friends like Max Graf had either left or were just about to leave the ranks of the orthodox. Freud was a man with a pen which fitted naturally into his hand, but the situation, he felt, called for a sword.

It is true that he had not taken Adler's and Jung's departure lying down. But he had contented himself with demolishing them by what he wrote, not by the way he acted. Even this literary aggression, however, was more than he felt comfortable with. He decided, after his outburst in the Nuremburg hotel, not to dignify his detractors, critics and "enemies" by answering them directly. The man whose first boyhood heroes had been warriors, from that time on shunned open argument, controversy and polemics. He avoided all opportunity for public discussion of his doctrine and for rebuttal with his critics. Not once, in all the years he was under attack, did he defend himself directly. Moreover, he advised his followers to do the same: to answer criticism by their positive accomplishments, and not to dissipate their energies in arid controversy. The only reprisals he permitted himself for the slings and arrows of his detractors were bitter little potshots at their points of view imbedded in his books and articles.

Time had thus wrought a metamorphosis in the man who as a boy had dreamed of force as the answer to insult and injury. As the head of the International Psychoanalytic Association Freud might better have been as direct, aggressive and straightforward as the realities of the situation demanded. Instead he turned in upon himself, as was his wont, grew bitter with no direct outlet for his wounded sensibilities, and came to magnify the extent and character of the attacks directed against him. Long after his work had won widespread recognition, Freud continued to act like a man who daily faced the dangerous fire of the enemy. It is unlikely that for all his conviction that he had fulfilled the Delphic injunction to know himself, he saw his refusal to defend himself and his science directly in this light.

Rather, with the Messianic conviction that grew in him as his conviction of rejection grew, he came to see his struggle with his critics as a battle between good and evil. And he found in the pages of Anatole France, one of his favourite authors, a mirror which reflected this battle and projected it as a titanic struggle between gods. In *La Révolte des Anges*, France had made his thesis the disavowal of warfare as an implement in the battle for the victory of truth. Freud read and reread the chapters describing the development of civilization as a struggle between the revolted angels and Jahwe-Jaldabaoth. The concluding passages of the book impressed him particularly. There Satan refuses to accept leadership and certain victory because he is convinced that in overthrowing the old ruler by force in order to take his place, he would be tainted by the same brush of cruelty and despotism. "War will produce war," France wrote, "and victory defeat. God defeated will become Satan—Satan victorious will become God. We have destroyed Jaldabaoth when we have destroyed in ourselves the ignorance and the fear. We have been defeated because we didn't understand that the victory is of the spirit, and that within ourselves and only within ourselves, Jaldabaoth must be attacked and destroyed." Freud not only urged his disciples to read these words of France's and to steep themselves in this philosophy, but he broke a long-standing rule never to lecture to a non-analytic audience, in order to tell the members of the B'nai B'rith of France's message.

Thus, when Freud wrote, in bidding farewell to Jung, that "men are strong so long as they represent a strong idea," he was thinking not so much of Jung as of himself. With France's strong idea that the ultimate victory is a victory of the spirit, not of the arena, he armed himself to fight the cause of psychoanalysis against the enemies and obstacles that beset it. The idea was a strong weapon, but it did not suffice to win the battle that raged within himself. He wanted to devote his entire energies to the development of the theory and technique of pscyhoanalysis, not to its administration. And he knew that his personal involvement in psychoanalytic meetings, congresses, and struggles for recognition in the universities and hospitals—in the whole organization of the discipline as a movement rather than a science—would divert the time and energy he needed for the pursuit of the analytic investigations that were as much a call as any minister's of God.

So he resented the responsibility he had forced himself to assume. The more he resented it, and the more he repressed the recognition of his resentments, the more compelled he was to compensate for it by overplaying his rôle as protector. The father of the psychoanalytic movement became an over-anxious, over-protective father. Just as he acted towards his own children with the rigid, watchful authoritarianism of a Biblical patriarch, so he acted towards his children in psychoanalysis. Helpful, patient and encouraging as he was, he nevertheless kept a wary eye peeled for potential delinquency even among the sons who clung to orthodoxy. It became a function of the international organization to see to it that every move away from the letter of Freud's findings was immediately identified as a clear-cut "schism." As the father of the psychoanalytic movement, Freud would stand for no nonsense from any of his sons. If a son wanted to contest, tone down, or dilute a statement Father Freud had made, off with his head! This need of Freud's to brook no opposition whatever, but immediately to impose autos-da-fé, was recognized by both Freud and his disciples. "I cannot stand the parricidal look in his eye," Freud once remarked of one of his followers.

Psychoanalytic orthodoxy, as it developed under Freud's anxious guidance, became rigid. The ritual became invested with a tradition as hidebound as any church's. The walls erected around the tight little brotherhood of the orthodox in order to shield them from a world opposed to them, at last began to shield the world from them. Lastly, so stern was the voice of the authoritarian father of the movement—so stern was *his* father's voice—and so unmistakable his unconscious attitude of suspicion and hostility towards all those who were not members of the analytic elect, that this attitude was inevitably assumed by the brotherhood. It persists even today among orthodox Freudians as the spiritual climate in which they live and work. As Roy Grinker, an American psychiatrist, puts it, Freud's "living presence among the analysts resulted in a continued recapitulation of an attitude based on Freud's own experiences during the development of psychoanalysis, like a religious ritual the meaning of which had long been forgotten and the necessity for it long passed."

Freud felt and had said that it was too early to make a hard and fast, strictly defined conceptual system out of psychoanalysis. Intentionally, he had kept many of his theoretical abstractions like libido, sublimation and narcissism loose and vague—because he was aware that they must be kept fluid in order to change with changing observations. He knew that his first formulations were groping attempts in the dark of an uncharted continent, and that they served only to bring a tentative order into the chaos that had existed only shortly before. He himself recognized the shortcoming of his theorizing, and painstakingly and consistently worked on their improvement.

When he spoke this way, with the voice of reason, he spoke accurately and well. But his psychoanalytic children reacted not so much to what he said as to what he did. He spoke of freedom to amend, revise and change his doctrines, but the emotional atmosphere that he generated for his followers was one of rigid, watchful authority under which any attempt to deviate was treated as heresy. So his followers *have* interpreted every tentative word he wrote as the ultimate crystallization of God-given truth. A pedantic and strictly defined conceptual system is exactly what has grown up among orthodox Freudians around the body of Freudian literature.

11

War Outside, War Inside

Freud was not prepared for the war that shook the world in 1914. He was confronted not with the triumph or potential triumph of reason, but with its opposite: all those primitive, destructive, hostile drives he had spent his personal and professional life in combating and subjugating. What was the use of reason and his own lifelong dedication to its service if in the end man was still intent on murdering his brother? Must he resign himself to the recognition of a truth he had been fighting all his life—that man, despite the intelligence which differentiates him from the ape, is still a hopeless victim of his animal nature?

The war struck at Freud's fundamental convictions, but it also struck at his personal life. A son-in-law and two of his sons, Martin and Oliver, fought as citizens of the Austro-Hungarian empire, on the side of Germany. Freud worried about them constantly. Oliver was relatively steadygoing, but Martin, his eldest son, who had enjoyed duelling in his schooldays, skiing, and dangerous mountain climbing, was rather a reckless young man. His station as an artillery officer on the Russian front was by no means a safe one. Freud could bid him an unemotional farewell—a brief good-bye, and a hearty handshake followed by immediate resumption of the conversation he had been holding with the friend who accompanied him to the station. He could not, however, stop himself from dreaming that Martin was dead. (Nor, indeed, could he stop himself from seeking out and recording the wish that had given rise to the dream. That wish, he said, was "the envy of youth which the elderly man believes he has thoroughly stifled in actual life.") Martin and Oliver emerged from the war unhurt, but their father had died a little in the days of their danger.

Freud's own life and activities were restricted. International collaboration in psychoanalytic circles came to a virtual standstill. The ranks of Freud's favourite apostles had been riddled by war service. During the last two years of the war, Sachs alone remained in Vienna with him. Rank served in Cracow; Ferenczi and Eitingon were doctors in the Austro-Hungarian army; and Abraham, whom Freud dearly loved, served as a doctor in the German army in East Prussia. Food and fuel were short in Vienna. Sachs tried manfully to keep up with Freud's undiminished vigour for analytic discussion, but sitting in Freud's unheated study with him, both men muffled in hats, overcoats and gloves, he found his mind deflected by the rumblings of his empty stomach and the frostbite on his hands.

Freud's stomach was empty, too, and his hands frostbitten, despite his wife's heroic attempts to keep the household functioning as smoothly as ever for her husband's comfort. She saw to it that the tobacco, which was as necessary a part of Freud's diet as food, kept coming to him in uninterrupted flow, even with the rationing imposed by the war. Freud was a chain-smoker, his daily quota some twenty *Trabuccos*, small, rather mild cigars which were the *chefs d'œuvre* of the Austrian Government's tobacco monopoly. He was so addicted to smoking that he grew annoyed with men who did not smoke. Because of this, nearly all his apostles became cigar-smokers. Martha Freud and Minna Bernays used to set out for the tobacco shop where Freud traded, bearing the finest examples of their beautiful needlework. These they presented to the proprietress of the shop, whose gratitude took the form of extra *Trabuccos* slipped under the counter. Arrangements were also made with a Dutch analyst and friend of Freud's to smuggle cigars to him from Holland.

Smoking was so important to Freud that it even coloured his political opinions. Nearly twenty-five years after his deprivation by war, Freud told an American visitor: "Whenever the government steps into anything, it does it wrong. Take cigars, for example. Here in Austria we have a government tobacco monopoly and cigars are wretched. In Holland, on the other hand, where the government is not interested in tobacco—and the Dutch aren't heavy smokers, either—there are plenty of fine cigars. In fact," he added, "I have sometimes thought of settling in Holland for that reason."

His astonished visitor offered the opinion that Austria was doing pretty well with the post office.

"Maybe," said Freud, "but I assure you, if it were in private hands, it would not be less efficient. You must have an incentive. You cannot expect things to survive on empty idealism. A man wants to get something for his work. . . . To illustrate, I will tell you a little story. Itzig,' he said, "once joined the army—but he didn't get on. He used to stand around and neglect his work. The powder got wet, the cannon grew rusty and Itzig never appeared on time. He was lazy, but the officers knew he was smart. One of them finally had a talk with him.

" 'Itzig,' he said, 'you'll never get to be a soldier this way—the army is no place for you. You'll never get on, and we all know why. I'll give you a piece of advice—go buy a cannon and go into business for yourself.' "

As a schoolboy, Freud had been a passionate advocate of German nationalism. As a man, he told a visitor in 1930: "My language is German. My culture, my attainments are German. I considered myself a German intellectually, until I noticed the growth of anti-Semitic prejudice in Germany and in German Austria. Since that time, I considered myself no longer a German. I prefer to call myself a Jew."[54a] In spite of his preference, Freud's thinking, his writing style, his underlying dualistic philosophy, although they owed much to other influences, as we have seen, were markedly Germanic in cast. ("It is characteristic of Jews,"

J. L. Grey once said in speaking of Freud, "that they are most strongly influenced by the cultural tradition of their alien environment precisely at those points where their divergence from it seems most extreme.")[54b] The things with which he had identified himself as a German were things of the spirit—the places he loved, the books he had read, the literature of Goethe, the philosophic climate he shared with figures like Schopenhauer and Nietzsche. Now, with the war, Germany showed herself to be, of all nations, the most aggressive, the most savage. And Freud, Jew by birth, Jew by preference, was still enough of a German, even without his sons' involvement in her cause, for her rôle in the war to have struck at him cruelly.

By 1915 he had begun to write of "science's" deep embitterment at the loss of her passionless impartiality, and of the noncombatant's "disorientation" and the "inhibition in his powers and activities." And the recollections of the world he had known before the war and his communion with it moved him to one of those infrequent rhapsodic outbursts which serve to disclose the artist behind the constrained man of science. "He who was not by stress of circumstances confined to one spot," he wrote in a paper called *Thoughts for the Times on War and Death* in 1915, "could also confer upon himself through all the advantages and attractions of those civilized countries (whose borders had been closed by the war) a new, wider fatherland, wherein he moved unhindered and unsuspected. In this way, he enjoyed the blue sea and the grey; the beauty of the snow-clad mountains and of the green pasture-lands; the magic of the northern forests and the splendour of the southern vegetation; the emotion inspired by landscapes that recall great historical events, and the silence of nature in her inviolate places. This new fatherland was for him a museum also, filled with all the treasures which the artists among civilized communities had in the successive centuries created and left behind. . . . Nor must we forget that each of these citizens of culture had created for himself a personal 'Parnassus' and 'School of Athens.' From among the great thinkers and artists of all nations he had chosen those to whom he conceived himself most deeply indebted for what he had achieved in enjoyment and comprehension of life, and in his veneration had associated them with the immortals of old as well as with the more familiar masters of his own tongue. None of these great figures had seemed to him alien because he had spoken another language—not the incomparable investigator of the passions of mankind, not the intoxicated worshipper of beauty, nor the vehement and threatening prophet, nor the subtle, mocking satirist; and never did he on this account rebuke himself as a renegade towards his own nation and his beloved mother-tongue."[55]

Sophocles, Goethe, Moses, Anatole France, the gods of his own culture, represented for Freud the heights to which humanity can soar. But those heights were now obscured in the smoke of battle. The war threatened to leave a "legacy of embitterment." And it left Freud finally in a state of despair. But part of him remained the father of sons who were fighting Germany's cause: "We live in the hope," he was constrained to say, "that the impartial decision of history will furnish the proof that precisely this nation, this in whose tongue we now write, this for whose victory our dear ones are now fighting, was the one which least transgressed the laws of civilization—but at such a time who shall dare present himself as the judge of his own cause?"

From the abyss of his own disillusion with man's humanity to man, Freud dredged up a pitilessly disillusioned answer to the "Why?" of the war. Disillusion about the uncivilized behaviour of mankind is unjustified. Man's civilized behaviour, his altruism, his social adaptability, are at best illusions. "In reality," Freud consoled himself, "our fellow citizens have not sunk so low as we feared, because they had never risen so high as we believed." War cannot be abolished—"there will be, must be, wars." And if this is so, "is it not we who must give in, who must adapt ourselves to them?" He himself believed that life was a task which had to be performed. With the war, he projected this dour philosophy as an answer for all mankind. The concluding sentences of *Thoughts on War and Death* read: "To endure life remains, when all is said, the first duty of all living beings. Illusion can have no value if it makes this more difficult for us. We remember the old saying: 'If you desire peace, prepare for war.' It would be timely thus to paraphrase it: 'If you would endure life, be prepared for death.' "[55a]

Freud's own concern with death had inevitably been intensified by his father's death. This concern in its turn had led him almost as inevitably to the memory of the greatest literary personification of preoccupation with death—Hamlet. For Freud, to remember was to analyse. Long before the war which filled him with the awareness of death, he had psycholanalysed Hamlet and, incidentally, Shakespeare. He had done this first in *The Interpretation of Dreams*. He had concluded then that Hamlet was rooted in the same soil as Sophocles' *Œdipus Rex*. The theme of the two plays was the same, he said. The only difference lay in the treatment of the theme—a difference made necessary by the progress of the force of repression in the emotional life of humanity during the two widely separated periods of civilization.

Sophocles had brought the naked incestuous wish-fantasy of the child out into the open, and had clothed it with as much explicit horror as any anxiety dream. In Hamlet, the prototype of modern man, the wish to lie with his mother can only be detected by interpreting the symptoms which his layers of repression produced. Throughout the play, Hamlet hesitates to accomplish his task of revenge upon his father's murderer. Shakespeare stated neither the cause nor the motives of this hesitation, and until Freud turned his own Œdipal eye on Hamlet's dilemma, no one had successfully interpreted the reasons for Hamlet's tortured inertia.

Freud's answer was the answer to his own riddle. He said then: "Hamlet is able to do anything but take vengeance upon the man who did away with his father and has taken his father's place with his mother—the man who shows him in realization the repressed desires of his own childhood. The loathing which should have driven him to vengeance is thus replaced by self-reproach, by conscientious scruples, which tell him that he himself is no better than the murderer whom he is required to punish. I have here translated into consciousness what had to remain unconscious in the mind of the hero. . . . It can of course be only the poet's own psychology with which we are confronted in Hamlet; and in a work on Shakespeare by Georg Brandes I find the statement that the drama was composed immediately after the death of Shakespeare's father—that is to say, when he was still mourning his loss, and during a revival, as we may fairly assume, of his own childish feelings in respect of his father. It is known, too, that Shakespeare's son, who died in childhood, bore the name of Hamnet (identical with Hamlet)."[56]

Freud was enabled to make the brilliant deductions he did about Hamlet and about other characters he weighed in the same scales, because he himself had lived and was living the rôle. Within Freud's own heart, the loathing for his father existed side by side with "self-reproach," and "conscientious scruples" which told him that he was no better than a murderer. Like Shakespeare, who composed a masterpiece while mourning the loss of his father, Freud, at a time of similar bereavement, created the book which he and his admirers consider to be his own masterpiece. It is, he said, only the poet's own psychology which confronts us in Hamlet. Similarly, it is only Freud's own psychology which confronts us in *The Interpretation of Dreams*. In a kind of projection of his own tormented and unresolved relation with his father, Freud took to analysing Hamlet in place of himself. This, he practically admitted: "I have here translated into consciousness," he said, "what had to remain unconscious in the mind of the hero."

Hamlet, as a surrogate for what Freud refused to face within his own heart, persisted as a subject of thought and investigation for Freud and for his followers for many years. But soon he began, with the duality that was so characteristic of him, to analyse and draw .conclusions about the most constructive life forces as well as the nature of death. This force was poetic and artistic creation.

The problem of the artist and his creative imagination concerned him as deeply as the problem of the individual and his need for destruction; for the one, like the other, was his own problem. He found, after thought, that the artist resembled the neurotic in his withdrawal from an unsatisfactory reality into a world of imagination. But where the neurotic was rudderless and lost in his imaginary world, the artist knew how to steer among the shoals of the unconscious and regain his foothold in the world of reality.

The artist's creations, Freud said, "were the imaginary gratifications of unconscious wishes, just as dreams are; and like them they were in the nature of compromises, since they too were forced to avoid open conflict with the forces of repression." But they also differed from the neurotic's fantasies because they were both capable of arousing interest in other people and of evoking and gratifying the same unconscious wishes in them too. What Freud then proceeded to do was to study the relationships between the impressions of an artist's life, his chance experiences, and his work, and from them to reconstruct, in the manner of a paleontologist with a few fossil remains, the character and constitution of the artist.

In this work, as in his concern with Hamlet, Freud was simply investigating by proxy another and different facet of his own personality—the creative. By 1910, when he published *Leonardo da Vinci, a Study in Psychosexuality*, one of the strangest and most convincing ghost stories ever written, he had found another surrogate, another mirror of the inner struggles and motives which animated himself. The book was ostensibly an analytic investigation of the unconscious forces at work behind the phenomenon of artistic creation. It was that, brilliantly; but it was much more than that. Behind Leonardo, who personified enigmatically the spontaneous intellectual rebirth which pervaded the world during the Renaissance, Freud saw himself. Leonardo, like Freud, was a complex discoverer. Like Freud, he was pulled all his life between the two opposing poles of art and science. Like Freud, he was consumed by an overwhelming need to know everything and the causes of everything. Leonardo resembled Freud in his belief in reason and rationality. Both men poured all their passion into the work which was their life. Because of such similarities between the analyst and his subject, what Freud wrote about Leonardo is almost invariably as true of himself as it was of da Vinci.

Leonardo left many notes and records testifying to the development of his intellectual life; but he left little or no direct record of his personal life. From the mass of notes describing nature, which Leonardo had haphazardly set down, Freud unearthed the one childhood memory he had ever recorded. Buried in a careful description of the flight of the vulture, Leonardo had written: "It seems that it had been destined before that I should occupy myself so thoroughly with the vulture, for it comes to my mind as a very early memory, when I was still in the cradle, that a vulture came down to me, opened my mouth with his tail and struck me many times with his tail against my lips."[57]

On the cornerstone of this disguised nursling fantasy, Freud added the few bricks of the known physical facts of Leonardo's childhood: his illegitimate birth, and the fact that he was reared by his mother alone for the first five years or so of his life, and then removed to his father's home and the care of a stepmother. From this flimsy material and through his own imagination and intuitive insight, Freud wrought so convincing a reconstruction of Leonardo's emotional development that it is difficult to believe the man he evoked is at best a hypothesis.

Again, Freud's process of mirror-writing, by which he reflected his own image, was the core of his reconstruction of Leonardo. He began, for instance, by saying that Leonardo's greatness as a naturalist was united in him with the artist, and that although he had left masterly paintings, while his scientific discoveries had remained in obscurity, "the investigator in him . . . never quite left the artist." ("In Freud's mentality," Wittels once wrote, "the mystical gift of the seer is continuously at war with the need for mechanical description. . . . He is afraid of his own supreme talents, and throughout his life as an investigator he has been imposing a curb on himself. One who by temperament is a seer has been ardently devoting himself to the study of exact science by the ordinary methods of scientific investigation.")[58] A little later, Freud points out that in the second half of Leonardo's life his interest turned from his art to science. Again, with the emphasis on the two interests reversed, there is the striking parallel of the switch in interest in Freud's own interests in the second period of *his* life: the switch from a primary concern with the observable clinical details of his science to a concern with the philosophical, theoretical overtones of his observations. It was this change which caused some critics to charge that psychoanalysis is no science at all, but an art form.

The fact, says Freud, that Leonardo passed the first years of his life alone with his mother "must have been a most decisive influence on the formation of his inner life. . . . Under the effect of this constellation it could not have been otherwise than that the child who in his young life encountered one problem more than other children, should have begun to ponder very passionately over this riddle and thus should have become an investigator early in life. For he was tortured by the great questions: where do children come from and what has the father to do with their origin?"[59]

So Freud led his readers back to the Œdipal theme. For under the tortured face of the childish Leonardo, who encountered one problem more than other children, we see the similar face of Sigmund Freud who, as a child, also encountered the problem of his family relationships scrambled in such a fashion that he must have greeted the word "incest," when he came across it, with a shock of recognition. In the relationship of Leonardo to his mother, Freud draws another implicit parallel with himself. If the infant Freud did not enjoy the same exclusive possession of his mother that Leonardo did, he at least enjoyed a spiritual conviction of exclusive possession—of being favoured and treasured over the other children in the family. Very early in his writing career he had observed that the child who has been the mother's favourite carries through life a conviction of success which frequently induces actual success. For the rest of his life, Freud would repeat this observation. In 1917, he used it as the closing paragraph of a paper on another hero—Goethe. There he said: "I have . . . already declared elsewhere that he who has been the undisputed darling of his mother retains throughout life that victorious feeling, that confidence in ultimate success, which not seldom brings actual success with it. And a saying such as 'My strength has its roots in my relation to my mother' might well have been put at the head of Goethe's autobiography."[60] Thus, like a child who repeats a magic formula in order to reassure himself, Freud repeated the magic theme—"my strength springs from my mother, from the well-springs of eternal nature"—not only in relation to himself, but in relation to all the heroes with whom he identified himself.

The mothers themselves Freud saw hardly as individuals, but primarily as vessels fulfilled by fate. For the personal sufferings of Leonardo's peasant mother, Caterina, Freud had no word. He said only that it was evident that she pampered her little bastard, and that in a manner comparable to his own mother's, she "brought to the world the noble son who was destined to paint, investigate and suffer."

The suffering, in Freud's Œdipus-blinded eyes, stemmed of course from Leonardo's father. The mother in the landscape of the Œdipus complex is a kind of gently rolling pasture upon which the infant gambols. The father is the fateful disturber of the peace—the God who is possessing the mother has the power to rend the skies asunder and blight the pastoral comfort the mother has created. Freud said of Leonardo: "He who as a child desires his mother cannot help wishing to put himself in his father's place, to identify himself with him in his fantasy and later make it his life's task to triumph over him. . . . We hear that he (Leonardo) was fond of luxury and pretty raiment, and kept servants and horses, although according to Vasari's words, 'He hardly possessed anything and worked little.' We shall not hold his artistic taste entirely responsible for all these special likings; we recognize in them also the compulsion to copy his father and to excel him. He played the part of the great gentleman to the peasant girl; hence the son retained the incentive that he also play the great gentleman; he has the strong feeling to 'out-herod Herod,' and to show his father exactly how the real high rank looks."[61]

It is possible, Freud wrote, that Leonardo's imitation of his father hurt him as an artist. "This resistance against the father was the infantile determinant of his perhaps equally vast accomplishment as an artist."[61a]

"According to Merejkowski's beautiful comparison," Freud continued, "he was like a man who awoke too early in the darkness, while the others were all still asleep." Again the rays transmitted by the spirit of Leonardo are refracted in the spirit of his analyst. It was Freud who, with the publication of *The Interpretation of Dreams,* was accused of "disturbing the sleep of the world."

Leonardo "dared utter this bold principle which contains the justification for all independent investigation: 'Whoever refers to authorities in disputing ideas, works with his memory rather than with his reason.' " Of Freud, it was said by Sachs: "He absolutely refused to accept any statement on the strength of a higher authority. He had no patience with those who did such a thing out of intellectual laziness or cowardice or because they wanted to have it settled with the least discomfort."

Because Leonardo had decided to work only with his reason in an age when reason was largely ignored, Freud concluded that "he became the first modern natural philosopher, and his courage was rewarded by an abundance of cognitions and anticipations; since the Greek period he was the first to investigate the secrets of nature, relying entirely on his observation and his own judgment. But when he learned to depreciate authority and to reject the imitation of the 'ancients' and constantly pointed to the study of nature as the source of all wisdom, he only repeated in the highest sublimation attainable to man that which had already obtruded itself on the little boy who surveyed the world with wonder. To re-translate the scientific abstractions into concrete individual experiences, we would say that the 'ancients' and authority only corresponded to the father, and nature again became the tender mother who nourished him. While in most human beings today, as in primitive times, the need for a support of some authority is so imperative that their world becomes shaky when their support is menaced, Leonardo alone was able to exist without such support."

Freud in his own era was able to exist without such support. He was, if not the first modern natural philosopher, the first modern psychologist to revert to the study of man's nature from within. He investigated not the secrets of nature, but the secrets of human nature. His courage to stand alone was also rewarded with a wealth of "cognitions and anticipations." He, too, relied "entirely on his observation and his own judgment." As a young man listening spellbound to Goethe's essay being read aloud, he had recognized "nature as the source of all wisdom." Like Leonardo, he had accepted the wafer and diverted the whole of his energies to "the highest sublimation attainable to man."

12

Old Man of the Horde

Reason was the god of Sigmund Freud's conscious mind, as it was the god of Leonardo da Vinci's. Under that conscious layer, however, there fermented and brewed in him all the needs, drives and instincts that have driven men to other than rational gods. It was inevitable, therefore, that a man of Freud's insistently analytic temper should eventually be concerned with religion.

It has not been difficult to understand the compound of repulsion and attraction Freud felt for religion. He hated the religion he had been born into because it had in his eyes made a victim of his father, and consequently of himself. Despite his admitted lack of faith, he had taken a stand as a Jew with the Jews of his community. Nevertheless, religion still represented irrational values which he had opposed throughout his career.

In Shakespeare and in Leonardo he had seen artistic creation in one of its aspects as the result of a compulsion to deny and triumph over the father, and to atone for the guilt of that triumph. Now Freud began to see the origins of religion in the same light. Three years before the book on Leonardo appeared, Freud had noted "a remarkable similarity" between obsessive acts and religious practices or ritual. He had described the obsessional neurosis as a distorted private religion, and religion as a kind of universal obsessional neurosis.

During the next five years Jung, on his own, was noting some widespread analogies between the rationalizations of neurotics and those of primitive peoples. Freud pondered and synthesized his and Jung's findings, and by 1910, when he published the Leonardo paper, he was saying that psychoanalysis had shown the intimate connection between the father complex and belief in God. He held that the personal God of an individual is nothing but the psychological equivalent of an exalted image of the father. Almighty God and kindly nature are simply sublimations of father and mother, or rather, "revivals and restorations" of the infantile conceptions of both parents, he said. "Religiousness," he concluded, "is biologically traced to the long period of helplessness and need of help of the little child. When the child grows up and realizes his loneliness and weakness in the presence of the great forces of life, he then perceives his condition as in childhood and seeks to disavow his despair through a regressive revival of the protecting forces of childhood."[62]

In 1912, two years after his look at Leonardo had inspired these words, he published his first integrated investigation into the psychology of religion, *Totem and Taboo*. In it Freud undertook to explain the psychological basis of Christianity and of all forms of organized religion by bringing it within the orbit of the Œdipus complex. He began by pointing out that the dread of incest was even more demonstrable and closer to the surface among primitive peoples than it is among civilized races, and that this dread had given rise to certain taboos, or measures of defense against it. These taboos, in which Freud discovered the first form of moral restrictions, he examined in relation to totemism, the first primitive system of tribal organization, in which the rudimentary beginnings of social order were united with religious ceremonial. In totemism, as Freud had learned from Frazer's works, the worshipped being is always an animal from which the tribe claims descent. Freud felt it to be evident that every race, including the most highly civilized, had at one time passed through a stage of totemism.

The two most universal taboo restrictions of totemism

were the injunction not to kill the totem, and not to have sexual relations with any woman of the same totem-clan. In these restrictions Freud saw what he called "a striking correspondence" with the motor of the Œdipus complex—the desire to kill the father and to marry the mother. He therefore concluded that the totem animal stood as a symbol of the father in the primitive mind, and offered as supporting evidence for this theory the fact that the primitive tribes honoured the totem animal explicitly as the forefather of the clan. He also cited the fact, garnered from psychoanalytic observation, that children who developed animal phobias were often substituting the animal for the father, a displacement of fear common to the working-out of the Œdipus complex.

With this established, Freud proceeded to describe the totem feast, which formed an integral part of the totemistic religion. Once a year the totem animal, at all other times regarded as untouchable and inviolably sacred, was solemnly and ceremoniously killed and eaten in the presence of the assembled clan. When the mourning period had been sufficiently observed, a great festival took place. This description of the totem feast and its importance Freud had gathered from *The Religion of the Semites,* by W. Robertson Smith. Now he took into account, too, the work of Charles Darwin. He recalled Darwin's conjecture that originally men had lived in hordes, each horde dominated by a single, powerful, violent, suspicious man.

From all these component elements, Freud says, "there rose before me . . . the following hypothesis, or, I would rather say, vision."

"The father of the primal horde," he wrote, "since he was an unlimited despot, had seized all the women for himself; his sons, being dangerous to him as rivals, had been killed or driven away. One day, however, the sons came together and united to overwhelm, kill and devour their father who had been their enemy but also their ideal. After the deed they were unable to take over their heritage since they stood in one another's way. Under the influence of failure and regret they learned to come to an agreement among themselves; they banded themselves into a clan of brothers by the help of the ordinances of totemism, which aimed at preventing a repetition of such a deed, and they jointly undertook to forego the possession of the women on whose account they had killed their father. They were then driven to finding strange women, and this was the origin of the exogamy which is so closely bound up with totemism. The totem feast was the commemoration of the fearful deed, from which sprang man's sense of guilt (or 'original sin') and which was the beginning, at once, of social organization, of religion, and of ethical restrictions.

"Now, whether we suppose that such a possibility was an historical event or not, it brings the formation of religion within the circle of the father complex and bases it upon the ambivalence which dominates that complex. After the totem animal had ceased to serve as a substitute for him, the primal father, at once feared and hated, honoured and envied, became the prototype of God himself. The son's rebelliousness and his affection for his father struggled against each other through a constant succession of compromises, which sought on the one hand to atone for the act of parricide and on the other to consolidate the advantages it had brought. This view of religion throws a particularly clear light upon the psychological basis of Christianity, in which, it may be added, the ceremony of the totem feast still survives, with but little distortion, in the form of communionism."[63]

Freud's "vision" of the cathedral of organized religion rising from the swamp of man's dark need to expiate the blood-guilt of parricide was as immediately distasteful and emotionally unacceptable to the world at large as was his theory of sexuality. It did much to crystallize the impression of Freud, among his enraged detractors, as a monster compounded of one part satyr, one part Antichrist, one part Bacchus and one part Lucifer. There were those, however, who have found validity in the insight which gave it breath. For Thomas Mann, *Totem and Taboo* opened up "for the reader interested in the questions confronting mankind, a boundless perspective and [threw] light into the spiritual past, the early historical and prehistorical moral, social and mystical depths of human development."

In spite of Mann's judgment, this view of the religious impulse, which Freud was never to relinquish but only to augment and embroider, left no room for the inclusion of any of the positive elements which have entered into man's need for religion. Freud saw the religious impulse as a purely negative and fear-ridden drive, based not on love but on guilt; not on faith but on the need to atone; not on communion with a loved image but on anxious pacification of a hated figure.

The ideas he set forth in *Totem and Taboo* had been simmering in Freud's mind for many years. But he finished the book and published it in 1912, the year in which Jung and the Zürichers withdrew from the clan and set up their own totem. It may simply have been coincidence that Freud himself in his situation acted in a manner resembling the old man of the horde. Or it may have been one of those bits of psychic irony which characterized his life. But it is more likely that these assumptions of Freud's, like all his assumptions, arose out of the spiritual climate of his own life. The old man of the horde as he emerged from the pages of *Totem and Taboo* was an all-powerful, jealous, domineering, wilful father who imposed his dictates on his sons, ruled the roost with a will of iron and was murdered for his pains. Freud in this savage rôle might seem miscast. But to Wilhelm Stekel, who left the clan shortly before Jung, he did not seem so. Stekel saw in Freud "the primitive horde complex." For him, Freud was the Old Man afraid of his disciples. And indeed, the behaviour of the faithful Viennese sons in the Nuremberg hotel had to some extent justified the Old Man's anxiety. They accused him of being simultaneously ruthless and simple-minded. Freud in his turn had acted like a man whose life was threatened. "We are all in danger. They won't leave me a coat to my back," he had shouted. "The Swiss will save us—will save me and all of you as well." Towards his faithful Viennese sons he had maintained an attitude which—although it might have been commensurate with their abilities—was nevertheless reminiscent of the primitive Old Man. They were "crapule." They could not be permitted the dignity and maturity of self-determination. Of Adler, after his secession, Freud had made in private conversation a typically Old Man remark: "I have made a pygmy great," he said.

There is no doubt that Freud's concept of the origins of religion in general arose out of the conditions of his life. His father was one of these conditions. But his own unconsciously hated, consciously affirmed Judaism was just as important a determining factor. In his theoretical writing about religion, Freud acted as if he had a need not only to deny and reject the religion he had been born into, but all religion.

It was the Christian world which had oppressed Freud and set him apart as an alien. It therefore seems only psychologically fitting that he should have drawn parallels between Christianity and the primitive attitudes. In reality, however, his attitude towards the Christian world was not quite so simple. He hated his Christian oppressors, as he had every emotional right to do. But he also, like every Jew who has been set apart, yearned unconsiously to become a part of their world.

Freud had a passion for travel. Particularly, he loved to visit the cities and places of the ancient world. Of all these places, it was Rome which he most yearned to see. This yearning had begun when as a boy he had dreamed of Hannibal, the great Semitic general, who had longed, too, to see and conquer Rome. When Freud embarked upon his hero-worship, he appropriated Hannibal's wish.

Although he soon outgrew his childish hero-worship, he never relinquished the wish. When, as a man of more than forty, he wrote *The Interpretation of Dreams*, he discussed a series of dreams which centered about his longing to visit Rome. It might have been expected that his interests would have led him to prefer Greece, for example, with its greater heritage of philosophic and artistic vitality. In *The Interpretation of Dreams*, however, he gives the clue to the persistence of his dream. There he called Rome "the promised land"; and there he said that Rome symbolized for him only one thing—"the organization of the Catholic Church."

His unconsummated wish to go to Rome reminded Freud, appropriately enough, of one of those pointed Jewish stories of which he was so fond. The story concerned a poor Jew who sneaked into the Karlsbad express without a ticket. The conductor soon learned that the Jew was aboard illegally. At each succeeding call for tickets as the train progressed from station to station, he reviled the Jew more and more harshly. Finally, at one of the stops, the poor Jew met a friend who asked him where he was going. "To Karlsbad," he shrugged, "—if my constitution holds out."

And so would he get to Rome without the passport of Christian birth—if his constitution held out. Hannibal, he said in discusing the same dreams, symbolized "the tenacity of the Jews" in the struggle against the organization of the Church. Was his wish, then, a desire to penetrate the stronghold of the Church in order to conquer it, as Hannibal wished to conquer Rome? Or was it a wish to identify himself with the Church? These questions Freud did not answer. He wrote only two ambiguously phrased sentences in explanation of his sustained craving. "The significance for our emotional life," he said, "which the anti-Semitic movement has since assumed, helped to fix the thoughts and impressions of those early days. Thus the desire to go to Rome has in my dream-life become the mask and symbol for a number of warmly cherished wishes, for whose realization one had to work with the tenacity and singlemindedness of the Punic general, though their fulfilment at times seemed as remote as Hannibal's lifelong wish to enter Rome."[64]

Attracted irresistibly towards Rome, the seat of the Church, Freud nevertheless took a Hannibal-like revenge on it in *Totem and Taboo* by implying that all of its high-flown Christian virtues were based on parricide, blood-guilt, fear and hate. Whatever the secret content of the "number of warmly cherished wishes" of which he spoke, workers in the analytic vineyard have attempted to prove that Freud's desire to enter Rome was a desire to enter the Church, to penetrate for himself its shrine and fountainhead, and to identify himself finally and peacefully with his oppressors.

Freud himself either cut short the interpretation of his dreams about Rome or veiled them in such obscurity and ambiguity that it is difficult to decipher what he really thought they meant. One analytic worker, however, recently undertook to reinterpret these dreams of Freud's. For him, they are all expressions of Freud's unconscious wish to feel free to adopt Christianity. The most important determining factor of all Freud's dreams, in his view, is Freud's inner struggle for unhampered advancement; in order for this to be accomplished, Freud unconsciously felt that he "would have to conclude a Faustian pact—he would have to sell his soul to the Church."[65] In the dreams about Rome and in other dreams, the theme of baptism continually crops up, he maintains, and this shows clearly that Freud all through his life wanted to demand the same privileges as a Christian. Freud felt alone, as he well might have, in his struggle for existence and recognition. He is the poor Jew who has no ticket on the train to Karlsbad although all the other passengers are riding legally. Freud dreams of hell, and he means that hell on earth is the destiny of the Jews.

In many of his dreams he is unable to walk; in most of them he is somehow hindered from the accomplishment of his aim. He might well have been saying: "I should dearly love to rid myself of this oppressive burden of Jewishness. I should like to walk free and unfettered as other men do. But I would be ashamed to deny my birth and renounce my ancestry, for if I did, I should feel even more guilty than I now do."

Another analytic writer[66] recently made the same point: that Freud unconsciously resented his Jewishness and repressed the conscious expression of that resentment. He quotes Freud's own emphasis of the fact that he had always had an intense desire to play the "strong man," the man who controls his own destiny, and says that undoubtedly the persecution he suffered as a Jew strengthened him in his conviction that knowledge and power would be necessary to offset the forces of political and social injustice. Then the realization that being a Jew made him helpless in the face of humiliation and discrimination was more than he could bear. It was undoubtedly the feeling of helplessness which his Jewishness engendered that made him unconsciously yearn for Rome and conversion. But this wish involved implications of racial and family disloyalty. Thus it was intolerable to Freud's strict conscience, and therefore it had to be repressed and relegated to his unconscious mind.

It is impossible, since Freud was so careful to veil the ultimate truth about himself, to prove the truth of these assertions. But there is good circumstantial reason to believe that it was the stern and righteous voice of Freud's conscience which prevented him from taking the assimilationist path of his wife's uncle, the apostate professor who became a reader to Ludwig of Bavaria.

Freud did get to Rome. For many years he had been restrained from going because its summer climate was considered to be unhealthy. But shortly after the end of his hopes for Jung and shortly after the publication of *Totem and Taboo*, the wish was consummated. It was in September 1913 that he made this first of many trips, and the visit, as might be expected from the content of his dreams, proved to be of great emotional significance. In Rome at last, where he had for so long yearned to be, he was impressed by only one thing: the statue of Moses which Michelangelo had made for the tomb of Pope Julius. In the birthplace and stronghold of Christianity, he sought and found a spiritual identity with a great leader of his own people. He would bind up the wounds of rejection and humiliation he felt he had suffered at the hands of the Calvinist Zürichers, with the stuff of the patriarchal robe of Moses—just as he had sought a general identity with the men of the B'nai B'rith after the rejection he had suffered at the hands of Breuer and the Viennese medical world. And he would find in Moses a civilized counterpart of his primitive Old Man of the horde: a wise, authoritative, dominating patriarch brought closer in time and spirit to the condition of civilized man. This Moses, like that Leonardo and that Hamlet, bore a strange and startling resemblance to a dominant side of Freud's nature. Whatever Michelangelo might have had in mind in creating his heroic figure of Moses, Freud saw in it a struggle and resolution analogous to his own. Never had a work of art affected him so profoundly.

Freud returned again and again to the "unlovely" Corso Cavour where, in the lonely, deserted church, the statue stood. He would mount the steps and stand lost in reflection before the stone gaze of Moses. Before long, the stone seemed to melt, and under "the angry scorn of the hero's glance," Freud trembled. Sometimes he crept cautiously out of the half-gloom of the interior "as though I myself," he said, "belonged to the mob upon which his eye is turned—the mob which can hold fast no conviction, which has neither faith nor patience and which rejoices when it has regained its illusory idols."

In this mystic contemplation of Michelangelo's creation, Freud found an historical analogue of his trial by the Zürich "mob" which neither held to his conviction nor had faith and patience with him, and which presumably rejoiced when it had regained "its illusory idols." This disguised analogue, which he incorporated into a paper called *The Moses of Michelangelo,* upon his return from Rome, he must have realized would be an easily decipherable record of his own emotions of betrayal at the hands of the Zürichers, and of his own resolution to stand steadfast despite the slings and arrows of outrageous fate. For *The Moses of Michelangelo* was published anonymously.

Never before, and never after, was Freud impelled to disclaim authorship of any of his work. The paper appeared in *Imago,* one of the official psychoanalyst periodicals, and it was prefaced simply by an editorial note: "Although this paper does not, strictly speaking, conform to the conditions under which contributions are accepted for publication in this Journal, the editors have decided to print it, since the author, who is personally known to them, belongs to psychoanalytic circles, and since his mode of thought has in point of fact a certain resemblance to the methodology of psychoanalysis."[67]

Others had viewed Michelangelo's enigmatic statue and had not considered it to be a generalized character study of Moses. They had thought that Michelangelo had intended to catch Moses at a specific and significant moment of his life—the descent from Mount Sinai when Moses, who had just received the Ten Commandments from the Lord, perceives with horror that his people are dancing about and worshipping a Golden Calf which they have made in his absence. Just so Freud had been the lawgiver of psychoanalysis who saw, not at Sinai but at Munich, his people, the Zürichers, bow down not to *his* word but to the Golden Calf of their heresy.

In Freud's opinion, Michelangelo had intended his figure as a character study. Into the stone face and stone body of the heroic figure of Moses, Freud read the character which he himself would thereafter present to the world. Michelanglo, he said, had intended to create an "image of a passionate leader of mankind who, concious of his divine mission as a lawgiver, meets the uncomprehending opposition of man." He found evidence, in the pose of the body, of "the conflict which is bound to arise between such a reforming genius and the rest of mankind." He saw "anger, contempt and pain" typified in this Moses—emotions which he said were inevitable to "the nature of a superman of this kind." He agreed wholeheartedly with a quoted authority who felt that Michelangelo had created a character type "embodying an inexhaustible inner force which tames the recalcitrant world." And he agreed with another critic who observed that the secret of the emotional impact of the work was "the artistic contrast between the inward fire and the outer calm of his bearing."

Freud came finally to the conclusion that, while the figure of the seated Moses seemed fraught with motion, he had been immobilized not at the moment, when he was just about to spring into action, but at the moment when the remnant of invo untary motion was still passing through him. For Freud had arrived at a conception of Moses—regardless of Michelangelo's intent—which fits exactly into his idealized conception of his own emotional state and its aftermath at the time of his trial by the worshippers of the Golden Calf. "In his first transport of fury," he said, "Moses desired to act, to spring up and take vengeance and forget the Tables; but he has overcome the temptation, and he will now remain seated and still in his frozen wrath and in his pain mingled with contempt. Nor will he throw away the Tables so that they will break on the stones, for it is on their especial account that he has controlled his anger; it was to preserve them that he kept his passion in check. In giving way to his rage and indignation he had to neglect the Tables, and the hand which upheld them was withdrawn. They began to slide down and were in danger of being broken. This brought him to himself. He remembered his mission and renounced for its sake an indulgence of his feelings."[68]

In this renunciation of the "indulgence" of his feelings—a luxury which Freud had hardly ever allowed himself—he found the true majesty of Michelangelo's Moses. Although the Bible records that Moses in a fit of rage did indeed break the Tablets of the Lord, Freud felt that his interpretation of a Moses whose hand was stayed in the heat of his wrath was superior to the historical or traditional one. He said that because Michelangelo had not allowed Moses to break the Tablets, but had made his wrath the servant of his reason, "in this way, he has added something new and more than human to the figure of Moses; so that the giant frame with its tremendous physical power becomes only a concrete expression of the highest mental achievement that is possible in a man, that of struggling successfully against an inward passion for the sake of a cause to which he has devoted himself."[69]

Freud drew conviction and strength from the image of the leader of his people which he kept locked in his bosom. The qualities which had always been a part of him became intensified. The longer he walked in Moses' footsteps, the more he winnowed out of his life all those human frailties, all those "indulgences" which might have made his life easier and happier. Michelangelo had made Moses into a superhuman figure. Freud's struggle for self-mastery, his struggle "against an inward passion for the sake of a cause to which he [had] devoted himself," became the dominant motif in his life.

His friends and followers saw this happen. To Dr. Brill, for example, who devoted his life to the propagation of Freud's doctrine, Freud's identification of himself with Moses was obvious. To Brill's mind, there was good reason for Freud's indentification, for Freud, too, was "a passionate leader of mankind, conscious of his mission as a teacher, as an expositor of the dark recesses of his mind. He too was confronted by the blind opposition of men."

Hanns Sachs also was aware of the parallel which his master drew between himself and Moses. He points out that Moses' wrath was provoked by the very people he had delivered from bondage, and that the people in their turn were led on by the High Priest whom Moses had chosen to be his mouthpiece. Moses' resurrection—the spiritual rebirth of his teaching—was left to the prophets. Freud, says Sachs, expected a similar fate. Years after his death, Freud felt, a prophet would arise who would proclaim the truth which had been rejected in his time. And Sachs saw in this resurrection fantasy of Freud's a theme which harked back to one Freud had introduced in *Totem and Taboo*. "Every great leader," he says, "every teacher of a new truth or a new way of living, had to be sacrificed in order to gain the ascendancy of his ideas by the resurrection, just as the totem animal when it had been eaten by the worshippers was mourned and then deified after its resurrection."

Other analysts have been aware of Freud's amazing spiritual assumption of Moses' mantle. Oehlschlegel speaks of Freud as believing that he was Moses' "modern counterpart," and of realizing "that the key to Moses' unusual success as a leader and lawgiver lay in his remarkable ability to control his own strong passions. And seeing in Moses a reflection of his own great powers, Freud gradually became convinced that self-mastery is 'the highest achievement which is attainable to any human being,' and that this highest achievement marks the truly great man."[70]

Adler had once made a remark for which Freud never

forgave him. Shortly before the split, when the battle lines were being drawn, Adler had shouted: "Let us investigate the psychoanalytic method and its investigators by means of psychoanalysis—if it is, after all, so infallible a tool as you claim it to be." To Freud, this was unspeakable *lèse majesté*. And yet, time and again, in his writing, in his conversation and in his actions, Freud, laid himself wide open to such a suggestion. Of the Moses paper, in particular, this is true. To equip Michelangelo's Moses with the emotional colour and content that was his own, Freud had to overlook one of the most enigmatic of the characteristics with which the artist had endowed his figure, a characteristic which, under ordinary circumstances, would have afforded him enough subject-matter for several papers.

For Michelangelo, curiously enough, in the light of Freud's interpretation of his work, had adorned the head of Moses with a distinct and unmistakable pair of horns—such horns as are common to classical statues of satyrs, Pans and pagan gods. In all of Freud's paper, there is only one mention of the fact that, lost in daily reverie as he was before the statue, he ever even saw the horns: He said: "No other work of art in the world has been judged so diversely as the Moses with the head of Pan." But he neglected to explain, or even to pose the question, why Michelangelo had equipped the man who personified the most civilizing influence of the ancient world with the most characteristic symbolic accoutrements of the pagan world.

It seems obvious that Michelangelo intended to convey by the contrast of the horns with the majestic, dignified, heroic figure the contrast between the dying paganism and dawning civilization—or more exactly, the debt which even the noblest of men owes to his animal ancestry. Whichever he meant, this contrast was germane to his conception of the stature and significance of Moses. That Freud, one of the keenest of intuitive observers, was unimpressed by the significance of the horns is unlikely.

There was a more likely reason why he overlooked them in his interpretation of Michelangelo's statue: they did not fit into his conception of his hero. For the horns symbolize man's baser passion, his primitive nature, his link with the beasts—attributes and circumstances to whose sublimation Freud devoted the whole amazing fund of his vitality. Such qualities were unthinkable in the character of the hero whose counterpart Freud convinced himself he was. It was just because he refused to discuss the horns of his alter ego, Moses, although he was willing enough to discuss humanity's horns in general in his work, that he came in the end to resemble not so much the living, breathing Moses as the cold, captured Moses of the lonely, deserted church in the Corso Cavour.

Moses, cried Freud, was *not* caught on the horns of his passions. Moses was so much the master of himself that he could shut his eyes to the fact that his head was horned. And Freud, in the image of Moses, carried his conviction to such a pitch that he acted as if he saw no horns at all on the head of his hero.

Freud had always been certain of his Messianic destiny. (Those who hated him—and there were many—have put it another way: "He was a pampered child.") But after he found Moses in Rome, the conviction came into sharper focus. Through the tribulations and ignominies of his professional life, it gave him support and strength. And he came in time to act as if he *were* a Messiah. He was a kind, a benevolent, a good man, but he was kind without softness, benevolent without compassion, and good without mercy. He behaved always on the assumption that his word could not be questioned, his authority could not be opposed. "What claims are to be made on us in the name of tolerance," he wrote in 1932, "that when somebody has expressed an opinion that we consider fundamentally false we should say, 'Thanks for the contradiction'?"

He himself was full of contradiction. But it was not until the end of his life that he revealed the one that was root to his whole conception of the religious impulse. When he was dying, brittle and ancient, and when the menace of Nazi anti-Semitism had grown to explosive proportions, Freud sat in his study and worked on a monumental analytic interpretation of the Old Testament. The theme he had sounded in *Totem and Taboo* twenty-five years earlier he proposed to enlarge, buttress and document from the pages of the Bible itself. *Moses and Monotheism* was the only published fruit of this work, for he died before he could complete his project.

He had first been struck with Moses as World War I broke out. And his last work, which again dealt with the last great hero of his life, was published as World War II started. For Freud, Moses was conceived in war and died in war. Another great disinherited Jew, Karl Marx, had seen war as the inevitable outcome of man's economic environment, and had created a world of his own in order to overthrow that environment. Freud, an almost completely apolitical man, who saw war as simply another manifestation of man's spiritual illness, turned back in upon himself when the world went mad twice in his lifetime. Both times he found solace in the inner contemplation of the best that humanity had produced.

The man who had found Moses in "the promised land" of Rome developed two major theses in *Moses and Monotheism*: the first, that Moses was not a Jew at all, but an Egyptian; the second, that ethical monotheism was not a spiritual achievement that could be attributed to the culture of the Jews, but an outgrowth of the idea of one God which the Egyptian Moses had brought to the Jews from the religion of an obscure Egyptian pharaoh named Ikhnaton.

The weight of evidence was not on Freud's side. Biblical scholars and authorities on religion had for centuries supported the traditional view of the origins of Moses and of the origins of monotheism. Freud of course had made a habit of departing drastically from traditional views. But because the reasoning in *Moses and Monotheism* is not as convincing as it is in most of Freud's work, it is apparent that for the first and last time in his professional life Freud gave way incautiously to the fulfilment of an irrational impulse. All his life he had sublimated into supremely reasonable achievement the primitive wishes and instincts he had watched dominate other people. But now, in his last years, cancerous pain ravaged him. Cancerous anti-Semitism ravaged his people and he, the Moses and Messiah, was expelled from his home of eighty years' standing, along with his people. His books were burned, his money lost, his publishing house destroyed, his children's future imperiled. It is not to be wondered at that the defenses he had spent a lifetime in making impregnable broke and crumbled of their own weight. The wish rushed into the gaping hole.

Moses, his counterpart, hero, and alter ego, was not a Jew.

Moses was, in the reality constructed by *Moses and Monotheism*, the illegitimate son of the Egyptian princess who had found him in the bulrushes. Thus, said the wish, Freud was not a Jew. And in the fantasy common to every child unhappy with his parents, he became a prince smuggled by unhappy chance into the household of ordinary peasants. The Jews themselves, his brothers in Zion and B'nai B'rith, were not to be credited with a great cultural achievement. That achievement belonged to the Egyptian Gentiles. Freud, become Moses at last, as death loomed, exile threatened and his brother Jews returned to a state of suffering unparalleled even in the days of their medieval torment, cried out in anguish between the still calm, still eminently reasoned lines of *Moses and Monotheism*. Like Moses, he implied, he was not a Jew. All this had nothing to do with him. There was some mistake. He, Freud, was a man of dignity and courage, not the butt of a paranoiac house painter. The fate of the common Jew was not his fate. He was a Gentile prince in disguise.

It took Freud a lifetime to spew this wish—one of "the warmly cherished ones" which Rome had inspired—out from under the carefully maintained *cordon sanitaire* of his defences. And it is unlikely that it would ever have emerged as clearly as it did if death had not been staring him in the face. For Freud, at eighty-two, was at last saying, as directly as he could, that he hated his father. He had said that the idea of God is a sublimated idea of the father. He had then, in *Totem and Taboo*, made the primordial father into as hateful a figure as any son ever encountered. He had gone on to link the need for religion with man's most primitive and horrible savagery. He would in later works call religion an illusion. But despite all the denial of religion which he had affected, the *coup de grâce* was lacking. He had not attacked the religion of his father specifically and by name. In *Moses and Monotheism* he did just that. He took from the Jews two great things which had traditionally characterized them: a great national hero, and a world-wide cultural achievement. These he gave to the Gentiles.

13

Day to Day

Little in the outer circumstances of Freud's life betrayed the intrepid adventuring of his mind, or the ceaseless warfare of his inner life. Had it not been for the intensity of his will to work, and the quality of his wit and intelligence, he would have resembled nothing so much as the typical German paterfamilias—middle-class in his ways, rigid in his habits, solid, sober, *sehr pünktlich*.

"Freud knew what it meant," said Sachs, "to be dominated by one despotic idea." Obedient to this tyranny, Freud stripped his life of colour, adventure, impulse, indulgence and weakness. "To the unobservant," said Sachs, "it may have seemed a cold sort of passion, since it never was embodied in big words, in emphatic professions or in emotional outbursts. Yet it burned with a steady and all-consuming flame. Like every other faith, it imposed on the life of the believer severe restrictions and regulations."[71]

These restrictions and regulations set the inflexible pattern of Freud's daily routine. He analysed patients—until such time as he gave up the active practice of psychoanalysis—from nine in the morning until the one o'clock *Mittagessen* which he took with his family. After lunch, he took his "constitutional," an hour's rapid walk. Refreshed, he returned to work, the first hour of the afternoon session being reserved for consultations arranged in advance. After that, work with patients continued until seven or seven-thirty.

After dinner his evenings were dedicated, with the exception of Wednesdays and Saturdays, to the same unvarying regimen of work. Closeted in his study, he pondered, he organized his material, he wrote until long past midnight. The man who disturbed the sleep of the world was himself an excellent, if meagre, sleeper. He went to bed usually around 2 a.m., slept instantly and soundly for five hours, and awakened punctually, albeit with difficulty, at the same hour each morning.

His attitude towards holidays was Spartan. Catholic Vienna might celebrate the many holidays on its calendar, but Freud ignored most of them. He disliked the interruption of his work for any cause whatever. In fact, during the Socialist uprising in Vienna, when the streets were barricaded with barbed wire and patrolled by armed guards, Freud was surprised and annoyed when patients failed to keep their appointments. He did, however, permit himself the luxury of a long vacation, unvarying in its duration. From the end of June through the end of September each year he left Vienna. At the beginning he would spend the first half of his holiday with his family in some Alpine resort or the Dolomites, and the second half travelling and sightseeing in Italy, or later in Athens with his brother Alexander, or his disciple, Ferenczi. Later in life, as his health failed, travelling became impossible. His vacations were then spent with his family in a suburban villa on the outskirts of Vienna, first at Potzleinsdorf, and then at Grinzing.

Freud did not exactly relax during these summer months. Although his clinical work ceased during the summer, he utilized the freedom and ease of this time for his writing.

During the winter months he went so far as to indulge himself with two evenings, later one regularly prescribed evening, for relaxation. Even those evenings were not wholly free of work. The Wednesday evening, while it was somewhat social in nature, was devoted to the meetings of the Viennese Psychoanalytic Society. When, after the secession of Jung and Adler, these were no longer held at Freud's home, his only evening off was Saturday. Early on Saturday evening he would deliver his lecture at the Krankenhaus, until such time as he gave that up. But he never stopped playing *tarock* with his three companions. He would occasionally vary this rigid pattern. Early in his career, Rank and Sachs would come to his house regularly for supper, followed by discussion and preparation of articles for the psychoanalytic journals. Later, when cancer attacked his jaw and the mechanics of eating became both painful and ugly, he permitted no dinner guests. He found time briefly on Sundays to visit his mother, who shared his love for card-playing, and who as the years passed had become a domineering, extraordinarily shrewd matriarch. His love of card-playing extended to solitaire, and he would take time off from his concentrated labours to sit playing it, with his legs high on the back of a neighbouring chair, his cigar clutched in his mouth. Mah jong, too, amused him. On Sundays he would visit the art museum and the archaeological collections; ancient Egyptian and Greek exhibits held a particular fascination for him.

The theatre he disliked in all forms. He went only on rare occasions, when such plays as *Hamlet* or *Œdipus* were given, or when a good friend like Yvette Guilbert was performing. Music succeeded only in making him uncomfortable. Social functions he ruled out of his life almost completely. While he made time to receive friends who were in need of help or advice, and while he made it a habit to visit them when they were ill, parties, visits, and evenings spent in desultory conversation did not exist for him.

His friends and family took their places in the strict pattern of his life only by giving in to his ways. Sachs noted that "the old friends of pre-analytic time dropped off; they did not disappear altogether, but the occasions for meeting them became rare and exceptional. Their place was taken by those who participated in his work—that is, by the circle of his nearest disciples. It is remarkable that his family—his wife, sister-in-law, and children—fell into line with the greatest eagerness, without a grumble."[72]

Within this immutable orbit Freud lived the years of his

life. Although, when his fame was world-wide, he could have afforded a move to more spacious quarters, he continued to live for forty-two years, until the day of his exile, at Berggasse 19, the crowded apartment above the butcher shop. When illness attacked him and operation succeeded operation, he was warned to give up his incessant smoking. He never could entirely break the habit that bound him. Although in America he had dreamed of prostitutes, he never trespassed into extra-marital adventure.

With these bare facts of this stark life, another of those paradoxes which so characterized Freud emerges: the paradox of the inflexible, narrow way in which his body walked the earth, and the rich, daring way in which his mind investigated the nature of that earth's humanity.

The man who founded the discipline which became the sharpest tool in clinical psychotherapy was himself, in the second half of his life, not particularly enthusiastic about its therapeutic benefits. For one thing, as the years passed he lost interest in psychoanalysis as a means of cure, and became much more concerned with its development as a body of theoretical knowledge applicable to the interpretation of cultural phenomena. He came, in fact, to think of the psychoanalytic method as a way of life, and he was more or less irritated with those of his followers who made extravagant claims for it as a therapy. While he formulated the basic therapeutic procedure of psychoanalysis which is still widely used to-day, he eventually became negligent of the possibilities the procedure offered.

His therapeutic success had gained for him very early in his career the reputation of a miracle worker. Characteristically, he minimized these successes and dwelt on his failures. At the turn of the century he had treated a fourteen-year-old girl whom he described at the time as "the most remarkable case of my latter years, a case which taught me a lesson I am not likely to forget ever, a case whose upshot gave me many painful hours. The child became afflicted with an unmistakable hysteria which quickly and thoroughly improved under my care. After this improvement, the child was taken away from me by the parents. She still complained of abdominal pains which had played the main part in the hysterical symptoms. Two months later she died of sarcoma of the abdominal glands. The hysteria to which she was greatly predisposed took the tumour-formation as a provocative agent; and I, fascinated by the tumultuous but harmless manifestations of hysteria, overlooked the first sign of the insidious and incurable disease."[73]

During this same period, Freud was asked to treat a young man who had lost the abiliy to walk after suffering an emotional shock. "At that time," Freud wrote, "I diagnosed his malady as hysteria and later put him under psychic treatment; but it afterwards turned out that my diagnosis was neither incorrect nor correct. A large number of the patient's symptoms were hysterical, and they promptly disappeared in the course of treatment. But behind these there was a visible remnant that could not be reached by therapy, and could be referred only to a multiple sclerosis. Those who saw the patient after me had no difficulty in recognizing the organic affection. I could scarcely have acted or judged differently; still, the impression was that of a serious mistake; the promise of a cure which I had given him could naturally not be kept." Freud had been reminded of this young man's case by having been called in as a consultant on a similar case. Hurrying off to keep this appointment, he had put a tuning-fork into his pocket instead of the reflex hammer he needed for his examination. What, he asked himself, was the meaning of this mistake? The answer he found was this: "You fool, you ass, get yourself together this time, and be careful not to diagnose again a case of hysteria where there is an incurable disease, as you did . . . years ago in the case of that poor man!"[74]

Just as all of Freud's positive achievement was created within the personal framework of his self-punishing and pessimistic nature, so he continued to develop the therapeutic technique of psychoanalysis despite the fact that he brooded over his failures. The crystallization of this technique took place in five distinct phases. In the first phase Freud used hypnosis as a doctor who treats physical ailments uses a purgative—for purposes of catharsis. In doing this, he made three basic discoveries: one, that hysterical symptoms are rooted in past emotional disturbances; two, that these emotional disturbances undergo repression from consciousness; and finally that although discharge of these repressed disturbances through hypnosis may give temporary relief, hypnosis itself can provide no lasting therapeutic benefit. So, in the second phase of his quest, he abandoned hypnosis and experimented with waking suggestion, placing his hand on the patient's head and attempting to reassure him that he *could* remember if only he *would*. This phase lasted for only a short time and was abandoned before 1899, as we have seen, because the recalcitrance of certain patients made Freud feel ridiculous.

Blocked in his attempt to talk the patient into divulging his secrets, Freud reversed his strategy in his third stage, and devised a means whereby the patient unwittingly talked himself out of his secrets. This was the method of free association which disclosed the unconscious mind of the patient while his consciousness was still in operation. Dream interpretation at this time became an important tributary feeding into the main stream of the unconscious material unlocked by free association. But again these new discoveries in themselves were not enough to effect a lasting cure. For Freud's interest at the time still remained focused on the reconstruction and emotional discharge of the disturbing symptom-forming past. And he did not see as clearly then as he did a little later that the recall and discharge of the traumatic situation was not the basic therapeutic problem, but that a lasting cure could be effected only through the re-education of the patient's ego in order to make him capable of dealing with emotional situations which had previously been insupportable.

In his report on "Dora," which was completed by 1899, but not published until 1905, Freud gave his first account of the phenomenon of "transference" which inaugurated the fourth stage of the development of psychoanalytic technique. "Transference" was the emotional reaction of the patient to the analyst, and Freud called it that because he saw that the patient transferred to the analyst the same historic neurotically arrived at emotions with which he had reacted in his childhood to the most authoritative figure on his horizon. Since the patient more or less relived his neurotic past in his relationship to the analyst, Freud gave the name of "transference neurosis" to this clinically induced neurosis of the present. In the working out of the transference neurosis, the patient gradually learned to deal with the same emotional conflicts which he could not master in the past, and which he had therefore repressed and excluded from consciousness.

The formulation of the concept of transference is considered by many to be Freud's most important technical discovery. While Freud, when he first described the transference phenomenon, did not realize its full implications, its significance grew until it eventually became the core of analytic therapy.

The working out of the transference situation, because it is a current, running re-enactment of the patient's pathogenic past, led slowly but inevitably into the fifth phase of psychoanalytic technique: the emotional re-education of the patient's ego in order to enable him, once the roots of his behaviour were understood, to cope with the present.

Freud arrived at his conclusions regarding the need for emotional re-education of the patient at about the same time that World War I put an end to the first period of his life work, in which his primary interest centred about clinical observation and questions of analytic procedure. After the war, he was more or less content to leave the development of clinical psychoanalysis to his followers. Once he had established the framework for the development of psychoanalysis as a therapy, he lost interest in its possibilities. Moreover, the war increased his natural scepticism about human nature and its ability to adhere to the banners of truth and reason. This scepticism grew hard and unyielding as old age and illness intensified his personal bitterness, until in the last decade of his life he seems to have lost faith altogether in the lasting therapeutic benefits of psychoanalysis.

Indeed, in a paper he published late in life, *Analysis, Terminable and Interminable,* he speculated about the posibility of ever effecting a successful psychoanalytic cure. And he came to the conclusion that "it almost looks as if analysis were the third of those 'impossible' professions in which one can be sure only of unsatisfying results. The other two, as has long been agreed, are the bringing up of children and the government of nations. . . . Not only the patient's analysis but that of the analyst himself is a task which is never finished. . . . The power of analysis is not infinite; it is limited, and the final result always depends on the relative strength of the conflicting psychic institutions. . . . We may say that analysis is always right in its claim to cure neurosis by ensuring the mastery of instinct, but that in practice its claim is not always justified. . . . A shrewd satirist of the Austria of old, J. Nestroy, once said, 'Every advance is only half as great as it looks at first.' "

He warned his disciples of what he called "*furor therapeuticus*"; he told the poetess H. D. in 1933 that "my discoveries are not primarily a heal-all. My discoveries are a basis for a very grave philosophy"; and he told an American psychiatrist, Joseph Wortis, at about the same time, that "analysis is not everything. There are other factors—the dynamic factors—what we call libido—which is the drive behind every neurosis. Psychoanalysis cannot influence that because it has an organic base. It is the biochemists' task to find out what it is, and we can expect that the organic part will be uncovered in the future. So long as the organic factors remain inaccessible, psychoanalysis leaves much to be desired."

Freud was in the last decade of his life when he made these observations. He was old and sick and by this time he must have been aware of the limitations of the equipment he had allowed himself to use in his search for complete understanding. He had armed himself only with the weapon of reason. "There is no other source of knowledge," he had written, "but the intellectual manipulation of carefully verified observations—in fact, what is called research . . . and no knowledge can be obtained from revelation, intuition or inspiration." Thus equipped, he had penetrated the irrational, chaotic depths of his patients' sick minds, only to meet again and again limits which he could not cut through with his single-edged weapon—the mystical, the extra-sensory, the extra-rational. It was, in short, the whole realm of organic intuition which he drew on so brilliantly himself, whose value in the search for truth he could not admit. "Some rationalistic, or perhaps analytic, turn of mind in me," he said, "rebels against being moved by a thing without knowing why I am thus affected and what it is that affects me."

His concern and his lifelong preoccupation was as much with the mystical domain of the soul as any theologian's or witch doctor's. But the map of the psyche which he drew made no provision for the soul. And while he charted a whole series of newfoundlands to take the place of the old country—the "id," the "super-ego," "the unconscious mind," and so on—he would never come to grips with the soul by name.

This discord between his scientifically rational approach and his mystical concern reverberated in his increasing bitterness and pessimism. For all his intrepid exporation of the soul, he was brought to defeat in the end by the limitations of his approach, by the things he was determined *not* to understand because they belonged to a world whose key he had pretended to throw away.

There was another reason for his defeat. He was, as we have said, his own patient. With all the intuitive powers at his command, self-analysis was not his *forte*. In this last decade of his life, he could not have failed to recognize that he had come to no successful emotional resolution of his own problems. It must have been evident even to him that he was an unhappy old man. It would therefore be surprising if he placed an inordinate amount of faith in the tool he had devised "out of his psychology"—for his own eyeing. Since he had been unable to fulfill the injunction, "Physician, heal thyself!" and since he realized the limitations of his therapy in treating his patients, he came eventually to regard psychoanalysis, in its therapeutic aspects, as a tool more fallible than exact.

When Freud told the poetess H. D. in 1933 that the reason she was not making better progress with her analysis was that "I am an old mán; you do not think it worth your while to love me," he beat his fists on the table for emphasis—in complete violation of the technical psychoanalytic rule that the analyst must be detached and show no emotion. H. D., indeed, was taken aback. "The impact of his words was too dreadful—I simply felt nothing at all. Anyhow, he was a terribly frightening old man, too old and too detached, too wise and famous altogether to beat that way with his fist like a child hammering a porridge-spoon on the table." The rule of analytic detachment—perhaps because Freud practised it so rigidly in his personal life—seems to have been a difficult one for him to maintain at this time. "He will sit there," H. D. said, "quietly like an old owl in a tree. . . . He will shoot out an arm, somewhat alarmingly, to stress a point. Or he will, always making an occasion of it, get up and say, 'Ah, now, we must celebrate *this*,' and proceed to the elaborate ritual—selecting, lighting, until finally he seats himself again, while from the niche rises the smoke of burnt incense—the smouldering of his mellow, fragrant cigar."[75] And, while his quivering patient could react to the irresistible force of his own personality with words such as "dreadful," "terribly frightening," "alarmingly," he could so far transgress the boundaries of the analytic situation as to intrude his own problems upon her. What, he asked her one day, was to become of his grandchildren?

Joseph Wortis, who went into analysis briefly with Freud in 1934, found him to be the same kind of exhorting, commanding presence he should not have been by virtue of his own theoretical standards. Freud condemned Wortis' manner of speech on moral grounds: "Mmmr, mmrr, mmrr," he said, according to Wortis, "you should talk more clearly. I think that way of talking is an expression of the general American laxity in social relations." Freud would sometimes give advice or commands, says Wortis, and "so far as analytic procedure is concerned, I did not find that the principle of letting the subject find his own associations was always observed. I would often give a whole series of associations to a dream symbol, and he would wait until he found an association which would fit into his scheme of interpretation and pick it up like a detective at a line-up who waits until he sees his man. . . . I wish to make the point that the procedure is far from foolproof and lends itself easily to pseudo-scientific conclusions on an arbitrary basis. A successful piece of analytic insight will continue to require the old-fashioned wisdom that good novelists have had for centuries. Freud had the insight, but I'm not so sure that the procedure he developed allowed him successfully to communicate it to others."[76]

Other people with first- or second-hand experience of Freud's analytic procedure encountered the advice and commands in a different way. Freud, they say, would exert a palpable effort of will during the analytic hour to prevent himself from advising or exhorting, but in the two- or three-minute interval in which he ushered them out, the barriers would descend and he would crowd into that time all the direct advice and injunctions he had successfully restrained himself from giving during the analytic session. Some were amazed at Freud's impatience with them; some by the fact that he used the analytic hour in his old age as an occasion in which to reminisce about the early days of psychoanalysis; some with his didacticism; some with his enthusiasm and excitement. When Wortis told Freud that one of his interpretations seemed to him to be far-fetched, Freud did not mask his displeasure. And Wortis found that he was frequently on the receiving end of disparaging remarks. When he protested, he was reminded by Freud that psychoanalysis was not meant to be a chivalrous affair.

But most of Freud's patients found much to admire in his analytic technique. For some, every detail of his appearance and gestures was noteworthy and remarkable. In these last years he analysed the famous and the infamous, but he restricted himself finally, when cancer had made savage inroads and speech was difficult and his daughter Anna conducted some of his analyses for him, to didactic or training analysis. Roy Grinker, the American psychiatrist, who went for training to Freud in the summer of 1933, saw him first at his villa outside Vienna. He seemed to Grinker remarkably young for his years, extremely energetic and active, with long fingers and hands which were in ceaseless motion. His hair was white and sparse, but his "magnetic" eyes behind thick spectacles were radiant and kindly. His manners were charming and "gave one a feeling of ease and security," and his questions were direct and searching. After two interviews with Grinker, Freud developed acute heart disease and pneumonia, and when Grinker saw him again after the few weeks' interlude which he allowed himself for recuperation, his physical liveliness was gone. He walked very slowly, the vitality seemed to have left his movements, and the next summer he moved only about the porch of his villa.

Grinker pursued his analysis at Berggasse 19. Here, after ringing the bell and waiting for a long time while dogs barked and growled, a polite maid ushered the analysand into a bare hallway and removed his wraps. . . . Suddenly the door of the sanctum would open and Freud appear. He first looked at the analysand and at his daughter's patient, then waved his hand in friendly greeting. He invariably grasped the outstretched hand only by the fingers and swept or pulled his patient into the analytic chamber. . . . Freud sat in a comfortable armchair, with a footstool for his slippered feet."[77]

Grinker found his speech to be low and almost incomprehensible, for by this time part of his tongue had been cut out. To emphasize his points in analysis he would pound the arms of his chair, and frequently the head of the couch upon which the hapless patient lay. When most intent and sufficiently excited, he would lean forward and loom almost directly over the head of the patient, "to whom," says Grinker, "his excitement was thus transferred." He seized with zest on details in associations and dreams. When names of places were mentioned in patients' associations, he would go into his study and ask to be shown the place on the map, which he would then peer at. "He had," says Grinker, "to understand thoroughly locations and relationships of houses and rooms, often asking that diagrams be drawn."

Although the poetess H. D. was frightened by the famous old man, she viewed everything about him and her analysis with him with a kind of lyric awe. As her analysis stretched into 1934, chalk swastikas began to appear on the pavement leading to Freud's door. But when Paula, the pretty little Viennese maid in a neat cap and apron opened the door for her, and she entered the waiting-room with the long lace curtains at the window, she found herself transported from the world of the swastika into a setting which was "like a room in Vienna in a film or a play." Havelock Ellis and Hanns Sachs gazed down at her from their frames on the wall. So did the "modest, treasured framed diploma from the small New England university," and "the macabre detailed, Düreresque symbolic drawing, a Buried Alive or of some such school of thought."

At her first appointment, she waited in apprehension for Freud to speak. He did not—he was waiting for her to say something. She looked around the room. "A lover of Greek art," she said, "I am automatically taking stock of the room's contents. Pricelessly lovely objects are displayed here on the shelves to right, to left of me. . . . No one has told me that this room was lined with treasures. I was to greet the Old Man of the Sea, but no one had told me of the treasures he had salvaged from the sea-depth. . . . He is the infinitely old symbol, weighing the soul, Psyche in the Balance. Does the Soul, passing the portals of life, entering the House of Eternity, greet the Keeper of the Door? It seems so. I should have thought the Door Keeper, at home beyond the threshold, might have greeted the shivering soul. Not so the Professor. But waiting and finding that I would not or could not speak, he uttered. What he said—and I thought a little sadly—was, 'You are the only person who has ever come into this room and looked at the things in the room before looking at me.' "

At first she was distressed by "the Professor's somewhat forbidding manner." But later she amended her opinion and decided that his manner was rather "curiously casual" and "ironic." To her, "his beautiful mouth" seemed "always slightly smiling, although his eyes, set deep and slightly asymmetrical under the domed forehead (with those furrows cut by a master chisel) were unrevealing. His eyes did not speak to me. I can't even say they were sad eyes." Sad eyes or not, she was reminded in the course of her analysis of a remark the Professor either had made or was alleged to have made: "At least they have not burnt me at the stake"; and of another remark that was made of Freud—a reference to his "courageous pessimism." She agreed from her experience with him that "he had little hope for the world." And he made, she says, only one request of her in the course of her analysis: "Please never," he said, "I mean never at any time, in any circumstances, endeavour to defend me, if and when you hear abusive remarks made about me or my work."

But within this framework of sorrow and bitterness she saw the tenacity of his positive purpose. She saw his great love of humanity, his pleasure and enthusiasm when in the course of the analytic hour some piece of insight had been gained or some crucial situation uncovered. "Striking oil," he called this, gleefully. And she found, besides his qualities of mind, which she summed up as "astute, methodical, conscientious, subtle, clever, original," qualities of character which had nothing to do with a forbidding old pessimist. He had, she thought, "so genial a nature, so courteous a manner, and so delicate a wit. He was easy to get on with, he could discourse delightfully on any subject at any time, with anybody."[78]

For nearly fifty years Freud kept a current, running record of those patients who interested him especially, often writing down word for word those portions of the histories which were particularly significant. Four of these histories were edited and published by him as monographs. Fragments and conclusions drawn from others can be found scattered through many of his clinical and non-clinical papers.

This analytic work and its recording would have kept a conscientious, diligent psychoanalyst busy, regardless of the quality of his work, for ten hours a day. But Freud's amazing productivity never faltered in the face of work which would have represented a full-time schedule for an ordinary man. In addition to his books and papers, Freud wrote thousands of letters. "On his writing desk," Sachs said, "he kept a big sheet of paper where, under the date of each day, he noted on the left the letters received, and on the right, the letters sent." He wrote with wisdom and vigour to friends, strangers, critics, disciples, patients, scholars, writers, sympathizers and enemies. He seldom failed to answer the letters even of cranks; and to his disciples he sent not only professional advice and encouragement, but help with their personal problems as well. Once Sachs, who wondered how Freud found time to keep up this prodigious correspondence, asked his family how he managed it. No one knew. The best answer they could give was: "He goes to his study and after an hour he brings us ten letters to be posted."

The letters, like the books and papers, were hand-written. Only on rare occasion did he use his daughter Anna as secretary. And even in the last weeks of his life, when the physical effort of holding a pen took as much strength as he could muster, he continued to write by hand. His handwriting was characteristic—large letters in Gothic script, the lines narrowly spaced and so close together that the words nearly touched. "In looking at one of the large sheets covered by his handwriting," Sachs said, "the first impression one gets is of an intricate network, a sort of labyrinth. On close inspection, it turns out that this labyrinth is quite readable; the letters are clearly traced, nothing is left out or neglected, all the little syntactical symbols are given with great diligence. The most curious characteristic of his manuscripts is one which Ben Jonson also noted in those of his friend William Shakespeare: 'In his writing he never blotted out a line.' "

There are graphologists who have found in Freud's handwriting evidences of his essentially visual imagination corralled and subdued in the interest of logic. They have noted evidence of his great energy and of the victory of his thinking over his feeling nature, a victory summed up in the phrase of one expert as "a man passionate in thought." Other experts say that his handwriting revealed a man who was a fanatic for truth, with no need for the confirmation of his ideas by the outside world. And still another is convinced that his handwriting showed him to have been a man of predominantly feminine inclinations, belonging to that type which Fourier described as "*femme par la tête et par le cœur.*"

With the same ease with which he wrote letters he wrote his books and papers, a body of work which fills thirteen collected volumes. These works, which appeared in a steady stream for more than half a century, he wrote, characteristically, without need to correct, revise or excise. He wrote them evenly, inexorably and without hesitation or pause, for he never set pen to paper until the thoughts he wished to express and the conclusions he wished to draw had thoroughly simmered to the point where content and construction were firmly fixed in his mind.

He never wrote until he felt a real compulsion to express himself, and he usually did not write until his ideas were ripe. "Then," he said, "it comes easily. When I have to write things to order—introductions and the like—it has always been hard." At another time he said that his conscious literary model was Lessing, and he quoted Lessing's dictim: "*Willst du schoen schreiben, so schreib wie du sprichst.*"

The fact that he rarely corrected a manuscript does not mean that he was not self-critical. He never rested until he felt he had established his ideas on as sound and broad a base as possible. This quality led not to the incessant revision of work in progress, but to postponement and sometimes cancellation of work already done. Thus, some of his early papers like "Dora," and his early books like *The Interpretation of Dreams,* were withheld from publication for several years while he repeatedly rewrote chapters. He disliked patchwork both in intellectual and human relations. He was never content to rest either upon insight, intuitive judgments, or his startling originality. As Sachs says, "If he found himself dissatisfied with the manner of exposition or considered that the structure of his argumentation did not stand up well enough under the weight which he had put upon it, or if he modified his opinion altogether, then he cancelled the whole thing and started to rewrite it. It made no difference if it was a short article, a chapter of a book, or an entire book." The difference between this attitude towards the formulation and exposition of ideas and the attitude of another kind of mind which is content to throw off sparks without causing a fire, Freud once compared to the difference between a casual flirtation and a responsible marriage.

Once, as Freud stood before the collection of Goethe's works which filled three of his bookshelves, he pointed to it and remarked: "All this was used by him as a means of self-concealment." He might well, of course, have pointed to his own works and made the same observation, for, as we have seen, it was always himself Freud wrote about no matter the shape and number of disguises he assumed. Freud has been called an *Augenmensch,* a man who lives through the eye, "born to see and made to behold," always perceiving the new in the old.

Freud's favourite reading was history. Rome and Greece interested him, but closer to his Semitic heart was the study of Oriental nations—Egypt, Babylonia, Assyria and Phœnicia. Archaeology fascinated him, just as the archaeology of the human psyche did, and he followed reports of new excavations with zest. He read, too, most of the world's great literature, not only in his own language but in English, French, Spanish and Italian, of all of which he had a full command. Goethe, who was the central spirit in the atmosphere of nineteenth-century German culture, Freud found an inexhaustible source of pleasure and stimulation. His life and works played a large part in Freud's conversation, and he is quoted frequently in his books.

Freud also read and often quoted Heine, the melancholy Jewish poet. And while it was the melancholy Dane, of all Shakespeare's characters, who most intrigued him, he had read and often discussed all of Shakespeare's work. With Russian literature he was also familiar. For Dostoevsky, whose personality he had analysed in a paper, he had respect, but little sympathy. Dostoevsky's irrational mystical world of self-torture repelled him, for it resembled the part of his own world upon which he had so resolutely slammed the door. He preferred by far the books of the "mocking monk," Anatole France, whose simultaneous disbelief in and fascination with the Church, whose lucidity and rationalism made him something of a blood brother, though France's graceful Gallic irony was far removed from anything Freud would negotiate.

Freud's prose style became an exact reflection of the qualities of mind and mode of thought that gave it being. Readers of Freud in English are handicapped in perceiving the fine quality of this style, although his British translators do him more justice than his American. It is a style radically different from the easy, conversational manner which made his lectures and social intercourse with him notable. An almost geometrical exactness, a Euclidian passion for purity was his chief aim in writing. But because his thinking was as complex in construction and as multilayered as a geological deposit, clarity was sometimes sacrificed. Thus his style, which gives a surface impression of severe logic and uncompromising precision, is in reality so tightly packed with meaning that a sentence read for the second or third time yields shades of meaning which have at first escaped notice. More often than not these compressed, complicated sentences read as if they have been poured through some powerful extrusion machine which has ground, pounded and moulded their component parts, before spewing them out.

To a casual reader Freud's style might seem cold and colourless. It neither woos the reader nor stirs him. It is largely unadorned, bare of flourishes, and has few seductive rhythms. He says what he has to say with boldness and perspicuity. He never reaches for artistry and he is miserly with imagery. But when the artist in him can no longer be restrained, and he draws a simile or writes a metaphorical passage, he sheds a rich light all the more striking for the sober setting.

Thus, in speaking of the deviationist analytic system which the Zürichers erected, he says, "As a matter of fact, they have caught a few cultural overtones from the symphony of life, but once more have failed to hear the most powerful melody of the impulses." Again: "Jung, by his 'modifications' of psychoanalysis, has furnished us a counterpart of Lichtenberg's famous knife. He has changed the hilt and has inserted a new blade into it, and because the same trade mark is engraved on it we are required to regard the instrument as the original one."

Trenchant statement and grace enliven Freud's style, although the complexity of his thought does give rise to elision and ambiguity. When Freud was confronted with one of his ambiguous sentences, he would reproach himself with having been guilty of *schlamperei*, a Viennese expression meaning sloppiness. And although literary connoisseurs esteem him as a master of German prose, Freud himself often said that his style was an example of Austrian *geschmeidigkeit*.

In any case, as Ernest Jones put it, "it seemed impossible for him to write the simplest sentence without infusing it with something of his originality, elegance and dignity. . . . It was these qualities, with the extraordinary purity and felicity of his phrasing, that led some Germans to esteem him as a writer, as others esteem him as a man of science."[80] His stature as a writer was recognized by the nation which had never accorded him any official recognition as a scientist: in 1930, at Frankfurt, Freud received the official accolade of German literary distinction, the coveted Goethe prize. Freud regarded the prize as "the climax of my life as a citizen"—although he added that the award reflected "the short-lived illusion that I was among the writers to whom a great nation like Germany was ready to listen. . . . Soon afterwards, the boundaries of our country narrowed and the nation would know no more of us."

14

The Passionate Will

Sigmund Freud has been bitterly attacked by the organized Church for his irreligious nature and for the allegedly atheistic influence of psychoanalysis; yet his own ethical creed and the tenets of his science coincide completely with the basic philosophies of religion. The science he had constructed preached the doctrine that instinctual drives be recognized as such, be known and made conscious, and then be turned towards civilized social goals. True of him, no less than of the creed of organized religion, was his conviction that the unruly animal passions must be tamed, curbed and sublimated in order to win personal salvation. Freud had preached that the forces of inhibition and repression were agents of disease; that only through self-knowledge could man fulfil his destiny. But, as we have seen, Freud never reached a complete self-knowledge. Repression worked as subversively within his bosom as within the bosom of any of his patients.

It goes without saying that Freud's morality and ethics were not the conventional morality and ethics of piety. He was brought up in an atmosphere of stern Jewish morality. High ethical standards were set for the children of Jacob Freud, and observed. It is true that this left its mark on his character; but the morality which Freud evolved for his maturity arose out of his dedication to his work, the work which he considered would lead an enlightened humanity out of the wilderness of its despair.

Ordering his life like a precision instrument, he believed that all men must so order themselves. He knew that he had sacrificed pleasure. "Science," he once said, "betokens the most complete renunciation of the pleasure-principle of which our minds are capable."

In order to produce and create at the inexorable rate he found imperative, he had to subdue the clamouring demands of the feeling side of his nature. Like a man balanced on a tightrope stretched between two opposite poles, Freud had to exercise constant vigilance and perfect control in order to maintain his precariously won position. This attitude left its mark on his family. The father maintained strict authority and insisted on complete domestic order, which gave the children little chance to use their own initiative, to make their own decisions, to learn a well-founded confidence through the lessons of their own mistakes. Perhaps because Freud's relation to them was more withering than it was encouraging, none of his sons approached the stature of their father. Obedient to their father's dictates, two of them at least, Ernst and Martin, became ardent Zionists. Martin, after a brief experience with the arts—he wrote a novel about his war experiences—settled down to the job his father had chosen for him, the management of the family firm which published Freud's works. When the Nazis destroyed the publishing house, the pugnacious and handsome Martin moved to London, where he now practises law. Freud's second son, Oliver, now works in Pennsylvania as an engineer. His third son, Ernst, good-looking, like Martin, and clever, is a moderately successful modern architect in London.

Freud's first child and eldest daughter, Mathilde, manages a dress shop in London. His second daughter, Sophie, died during the influenza epidemic after the first World War. And his youngest daughter and favourite child, Dr. Anna Freud, the only one of his six children who has made a serious attempt to fulfil the implicit parental injunction to immortalize the name of Freud, is a practising psychoanalyst in London. She has made important contributions to the science her father founded. During the war, in collaboration with Dorothy Burlingham, her close friend and co-worker, she drew notable conclusions about the psychological state of England's bombed-out children. She has taken up "the heavy burden" of the psychoanalytic movement, and directs the affairs of the International Psychoanalytic Society.

Freud, like so many fathers, had a particular fondness for his youngest daughter. Anna was interested in social work, and she became a school teacher, but she soon abandoned these careers to walk in the footsteps of her father. As her father's speech difficulties grew, she gradually took over his practice. Freud came more and more to rely on his daughter's help with the external affairs of psychoanalysis. Their common intellectual tie strengthened the bonds of their affection. Although all Freud's other children married, Anna never did. She has thus fulfilled the prediction her mother once made to a friend of the family: "Anna will never marry," Martha Freud said, "unless she finds a man exactly like her father."

Towards Anna's mother, the humble servant of more than half a century, "the poor Frau Professor" as she became known *in camera* to his most intimate disciples, Freud showed something of the same detachment he had towards five of his children. It is unlikely, with the amount of energy, devotion and passion he poured into his work, that he could have done otherwise. It was Freud who classified the basic nature of human energy—libido, he called it; *élan vital*, Bergson called it—as essentially sexual in origin. And it was he who probably first demonstrated to himself the transformation of that energy into what he considered to be higher goals.

He wrote in 1912, and he undoubtedly had himself in mind as well as his patients: "This very incapacity in the sexual instinct to yield full satisfaction as soon as it submits to the first demands of culture becomes the source, however, of the grandest cultural achievements, which are brought to birth by ever greater sublimation of the components of the sexual instinct."[81]

Freud himself left no more explicit record of his personal emotional life than Leonardo did. But his ideas about women in general are incorporated in the general body of his writing. Implicit in this work is his underlying point of view: woman is a breed apart and inferior to man.

In his earliest book on sex, *Three Contributions to the Theory of Sex*, written shortly after *The Interpretation of Dreams*, he had exposed in the interest of clinical truth his attitude towards his wife, and made some general observations about women which throw light on Freud's personal experience. He said: "The significance of the factor of sexual overestimation can best be studied in the male, in whom alone the sexual life is accessible to investigation, whereas in the woman it is veiled in impenetrable darkness, partly because of cultural stunting and partly on account of the conventional reticence and insincerity of women."[82]

In addition to her insincerity, woman suffered, in Freud's view, from her envy of the penis, an envy which Freud felt left ineradicable marks on the development of her whole character. He said, in a lecture he delivered on "The Psychology of Women": "One cannot very well doubt the importance of penis-envy. Perhaps you will regard the hypothesis that envy and jealousy play a greater part in the mental life of women than they do in that of men as an example of male unfairness. Not that I think that these characteristics are absent in men, or that they have no other origin in women except envy of the penis, but I am inclined to ascribe the greater amount of them to be found in women to this latter influence."[83] He was convinced that this penis-envy caused women to feel as much depreciated in their own eyes "as in the eyes of the boy, and later perhaps, of the man." Evidence that penis-envy never loses its sting he found in the mother-son relationship. "The only thing that brings a mother undiluted satisfaction is her relation to her son," he says, and adds: "Even a marriage is not firmly assured until the woman has succeeded in making her husband into her child and acting the part of a mother towards him."[84]

The sex act itself he regarded darkly. In *Degradation in*

Erotic Life, a paper he wrote in 1912, he said: "It has an ugly sound and a paradoxical as well, but nevertheless it must be said that whoever is to be really free and happy in love must have overcome his deference for women and come to terms with the idea of incest with mother or sister. Anyone who in the face of this test subjects himself to serious self-examination will indubitably find that at the bottom of his heart he, too, regards the sex act as something degrading, which soils and contaminates not only the body."[45]

It is hard to believe that so myopic a view of women and marriage was not influenced to some extent by preconception. He certainly considered his wife reticent and shy, and she may therefore have given him an impression of insincerity. If she did not feel "depreciated" in her own eyes, it is quite obvious that she was depreciated in those of her husband. It is also apparent from the emphasis which Freud always placed on his own relationship with his mother that his observation regarding woman's ultimate satisfaction resting with her son arose from his own experience. Martha Freud, whose function in life, whether self-imposed or dictated by circumstances, was to devote herself selflessly to the service of her husband and children, probably showed a freer and more spontaneous affection for her sons than she did for her husband.

Given the forbidding environment her husband created, and the limitations of her own natural inclinations, she could no more meet him on an equal footing than she could have pulled her weight in "a marriage of true minds." It was inevitable that she should have sought from her children the emotional satisfaction she required. It is also likely that since Freud saw her in the rôle of the devoted female, busily dusting the steps of the ladder of achievement he had climbed, he should come to interpret her selfless devotion and service as the attitude of a "woman [who] has succeeded in making her husband into her child and in acting the part of a mother towards him."

This attitude was, of course, not unjustified on Freud's part. But since he was impelled to marry a woman who would mother him, he unconsciously sought the perpetuation of that mothering which he had so enjoyed, and which he felt had so contributed to his success.

If Freud had not resented, as a husband, the absence of a more mature solace than that which the mother brings to her son, he would never have been able to speak of women as he did in old age. In discussing old age with a patient, as life drew to a close, he said: "There is an old saying that there is no virtue in youth. But it is just the opposite which is true. Young people are the only ones with virtue. The older you get, the worse you become. Women are especially awful in old age, but men are not much better. It is said that women are the best examples of love and human kindness, but that applies at best to young women. When a woman begins to age, she becomes an awful example of malevolence and intolerance, petty, ill-tempered and so on."[86]

A man to whom old age has brought tolerance, flexibility and acceptance does not project his specific dissatisfaction into a generalized denunciation of all womankind.

If Freud gained no real emotional satisfaction from his marriage, it was not surprising, for he could gain no whole-hearted gratification from any human relationship. Whatever difficulties marriage might present to a man who preached the recognition of repression and the necessity for a conscious realization of the rôle of primitive instincts in emotional life, Frued's marriage was not on its surface an unhappy one. It may indeed have been saved from unhappiness because the partners to it were too "civilized," too restrained and too "intelligent" to become the creatures of dissatisfaction. Certainly Martha Freud would never consciously generate a household atmosphere that was other than temperate and peaceful. And Sigmund Freud would never once swerve from the path of marital rectitude that grew from the seed of his general rigid morality.

Certainly he might recognize a momentary attraction to a young and attractive woman, as he reveals that he did. "In a friend's house, I met a young girl visitor who excited in me a feeling of fondness which I had long believed extinct, thus putting me in a jovial, loquacious and complaisant mood. . . . As the girl's uncle, a very old man, entered the room, we both jumped to our feet to bring him a chair which stood in the corner. She was more agile than I and also nearer the object, so that she was the first to take possession of the chair. She carried it with its back to her, holding both hands on the edge of the seat. As I got there later and did not give up the claim to carrying the chair, I suddenly stood directly behind her, and with both my arms was embracing her from behind, and for a moment my hands touched her lap. I naturally solved the situation as quickly as it came about. Nor did it occur to anybody how dexterously I had taken advantage of this awkward movement."[87]

He might again, as he once had in America, find his thoughts turning to prostitutes. And he might even write about an incident that involved them: "Once," he wrote in 1919, "as I was walking through the deserted streets of a provincial town in Italy which was strange to me, on a hot summer afternoon, I found myself in a quarter the character of which could not long remain in doubt. Nothing but painted women were to be seen at the windows of the small houses, and I hastened to leave the narrow street at the next turning. But after having wandered about for a while without being directed, I suddenly found myself back in the same street, where my presence was now beginning to excite attention. I hurried away once more, but only to arrive yet a third time by devious paths in the same place. Now, however, a feeling overcame me which I can only describe as uncanny, and I was glad enough to abandon my exploratory walk and get straight back to the piazza I had left a short while before."[88] Had a patient of his related this episode to him, Freud would not of course have rested until he discovered the unconscious motor of this "involuntary" repetition. But repression was so strong in him that this was practically the only "uncanny" experience he admitted having had in his rational life.

But never, even when a hostile world, resentful of what it believed to be Freud's "pansexualism," resorted to invective and called the founder of psychoanalysis "the Jew of Vienna," could a suspicion of slander be breathed against "the Jew's" personal life. Freud never deviated from the straight path of his righteousness, any more than he could deviate from the fixed character traits which gave rise to that righteousness. Conscience (or "super-ego"), Freud had taught, was the stern voice of the parent perpetuating itself in the child. Because Freud wanted to fight against the stern, commanding voice of his father within himself, just as he had wanted to fight the actual voice of his childhood, his conscience, stiffened by opposition, became an unyielding tribunal before which all the less stern, more pleasurable aspects of life were tried and found wanting.

Freud's face changed as all these character traits matured and crystallized in him. At thirty, forty, even fifty, his photographs show a man neither stout nor thin, tall nor short, distinguished nor undistinguished. His features were strong, virile, regular and quite handsome. But after the war his face became a sculpture upon which the record of his endless struggle for self-mastery was written.

Stefan Zweig, who revered Freud, described this change: "Now that his hair has grizzled," he wrote, "now that his beard has thinned until it no longer covers the firm chin completely nor conceals so effectually the sharp outlines of the lips, now that the bony structure of the visage has become more conspicuous, there has been revealed something harsh and unconditionally militant—the expression of an indomitable, almost mordant will." His earlier pictures, Zweig said, show "a glance simply contemplative, but now it is piercing and gloomy; the brow is deeply furrowed, as if with bitterness and suspicion. The lips are narrowed, tense, as though he were uttering an emphatic 'No' or coldly saying, 'That is false.'

"For the first time we are aware that a mighty impetus, the severity of a formidable nature, are manifest in the face, and we murmur to ourselves: 'No, this is not a good, grey old man, mellowed by the years, but an inexorable scrutineer, a rigorous examiner, who will neither try to deceive nor allow himself to be deceived. . . . A face that oppresses and frightens rather than one that liberates and charms, but none the less transfigured by the intensity of the profound thinker; the face not of a merely superfi-

cial observer but of one who sees pitilessly into the depths."[89]

After the war, Freud's work changed. In 1923 he underwent his first operation for cancer of the jaw, and thus came face to face with the propsect of his own death. In steeling himself to the possibility of the death of his sons in the war, in seeing all about him the wholesale destruction of life and of the culture that to him was the breath of life, it was natural that the philosophic aspects of his thought should become dominant. Now Freud, the analyst, became Freud the synthesist. The man who, by a passionate effort of will, had weaned himself from his natural inclination towards philosphy, returned, as death began to appear more inevitable than life, to his real career. In the closing lines of his *Autobiography*, which he wrote in 1925, he says: "Threads which in the course of my development had become intertangled have now begun to separate; interests which I had acquired in the later part of my life have receded, while the older and original ones became prominent once more. . . . This circumstance is connected with an alteration in myself, with what might be described as a phase of regressive development. My interest, after making a lifelong detour through the natural sciences, medicine and psychotherapy, returned to the cultural problems which had fascinated me long before, when I was a youth scarcely old enough for thinking."[90] Freud became, deny it though he might, a philosopher.

Deny it he did. "I am opposed to the fabrication of philosophies," he said. "I permit no philosophic reflection to spoil my enjoyment of the simple things of life," he told an interviewer in the late 1920s. In his *Autobiography* he wrote: "Even when I have moved away from observation, I have carefully avoided any contact with philosophy proper. This avoidance has been greatly facilitated by constitutional incapacity. . . . The large extent to which psychoanalysis coincides with the philosophy of Schopenhauer—not only did he assert the dominance of the emotions and the supreme importance of sexuality, but he was even aware of the mechanism of repression—is not to be traced to my acquaintance with his teaching. I read

Schopenhauer very late in my life. Nietzsche, another philosopher whose guesses and intuitions often agree in the most astonishing way with the laborious findings of psychoanalysis, was for a long time avoided by me on that very account."[91]

Freud offered what amounts to an apology for the course his work took. "A certain change has set in as regards the conditions of my work," he wrote, "and this will have consequences which I cannot conceal from myself. I used not to be one of those who are incapable of holding their own counsel about a reputed innovation for a while until it had secured confirmation. But in those days, time stretched bounteously before me; I had oceans of time . . . and the material which offered itself to me was so abundant that experience almost thrust itself upon me. Now, however, everything is different. The time to which I can look forward is strictly limited, and my days are not wholly occupied by professional work, so that my opportunities for acquiring new experience are no longer abundant. When an idea which seems to me new enters my mind, I am doubtful whether I can afford to await confirmation."[92]

Freud refused to apply the legitimate name of "philosophy" to what he was writing, and gave it instead the alias of "metapsychology." A partial explanation of this lies in the fact that psychoanalysis had already been dismissed by its detractors as a junk-pile heap of philosophic nonsense, and that therefore Freud was unwilling to lay himself open to the charge he launches against Nietzsche—"another philosopher" whose work is based on "guesses and intuition."

The fact is that at the core of all Freud's work, under the masses of detailed clinical observation, is the intuitive power, the "guesses" if you will, that set the whole scientific system in motion. Freud knew that the source of his intellectual strength and prowess lay in those natural gifts and inclinations which characterize every philosopher, and which in the end boil down to "intuition," "speculation," to the charge of "unfounded," "unproven" and "undocumented." In the mechanistic era of nineteenth-century science in which Freud was born, such values were anathema. So Freud clung determinedly to the method and spirit of nineteenth-century science. Thus, his century and his basic insecurity forced him to deny the sources of his own power, at the same time that he drew heavily upon that power to penetrate the irrational world of the unconscious. Although he charted the hidden ways of the dark world, he would never surrender to it. And thus, although he was a philosopher by natural right, he would never admit it. The unresolved strife of his inner life was thus paralleled in his professional life where the content was always at war with the form. As Waldo Frank has put it, Freud's work shows "a struggle between uneven forces, and the consequence is a psychological design that is drenched with the passionate and heroic will of its author."[93]

The "passionate and heroic will" expressed itself after the war in a number of works. The most important of these are *The Future of an Illusion*, which he wrote in 1927; *Civilization and Its Discontents*, in 1930; *Moses and Monotheism*, which we have already discussed; *Beyond the Pleasure Principle*, in 1920; and *The Ego and the Id*, in 1923.

Both *The Future of an Illusion* and *Civilization and Its Discontents* are essays which pick up the threads that *Totem and Taboo*, published fifteen years earlier, let drop. They are investigations of the origins of religion and morality, and they reflect Freud's now confirmed conviction that the events of human history, the interactions between human nature, cultural development and the precipitates of primeval experience, were no more than a reflection of the dynamic conflicts which psychoanalysis had studied in the individual.

By the time these books were written, however, Freud had charted another diagram of the individual's dynamic conflicts. He abandoned his original theory of the instincts, and arrived at a new and final dualism, stark and awful to contemplate. Back in 1911 he had drawn attention to the pleasure-pain principle in mental life, and to its eventual displacement by the so-called reality principle. He had dropped this line of investigation at the time because he considered it too theoretical and too speculative. But, in the early 1920s, he picked up this lost thread and charted his new speculative topography of the human psyche. The ego, man's consciousness, remained, and so did the id, or unconscious. But to these he added a third and new factor—the conscience, or the super-ego. The super-ego, he said, is the heir of the Œdipus complex and represents the ethical standards of mankind. It is the ideal towards which the ego strives and it is a pattern of behaviour and a group of standards taken over from the parents, which the child has incorporated into his own psyche.

Thus the influence of the parents finds permanent expression in the super-ego. But the super-ego is a troublemaker, for it functions as a conscience strongly tinged with the guilt and anxiety that cling to the Œdipus situation. Moreover, if the parents have been irrational and arbitrary in their behaviour, the child's super-ego takes on the colour of these attitudes. And finally, the super-ego makes trouble because the child has taken it over ready-made from its parents instead of arriving at an independent solution of the conflict between the pleasure and reality principles.

With the concept of the super-ego, Freud came at last to project as a scientific principle that inner voice of arbitrary authority which had plagued and divided him all his life. But again, the fact that one of Freud's speculative concepts can be traced back to the circumstances of his own life does not destroy the validity of that concept.

Along with the addition of the harassing super-ego to the structure of the psyche came Freud's bitterer perspective and revised view of the conflicts besetting that psyche. The original protagonists of this instinctual conflict had been the libido and the ego, the libido coming to represent not so much sex as generalized pleasure, and the ego identified with reality, or the demands of civilized life. But when Freud arrived at the concept of narcissism, the opposition between the libido and the ego had broken down. For if individuals could be in love with themselves, he had reasoned, then the ego itself must be in some part a love-object, and consequently be in league, and not opposed to, some part of libido.

Thus Freud sought a new polarity, and found one which was as much the outcome of the feelings that war, old age and approaching disintegration had engendered in him as it was of scientific acumen. The final polarity, the conflict between the life and death instincts, was announced in 1920 in *Beyond the Pleasure Principle*, when Freud was suffering from the shock of the death of his daughter Sophie.

Under the heading of life instincts, or Eros, as Freud called them, he included both the instincts for self-preser vation (which had formerly belonged to the domain of the libido), and for race preservation (formerly lodged in the house of the ego). Eros he contrasted with its bitter enemy, death, or destruction "which works," he said, "in silence." To Freud, with his need for discovering the motive power of all human behaviour, and with his passion for proving that all acts are purposeful, it now appeared that, since all beings die, there must be a will to die. How else, he asked, can we explain suicidal tendencies, masochistic behaviour, the striving towards Nirvana, and those impulses towards destruction, dissolution and annihilation that periodically motivate all of us?

The tension he propounded between life and death he visualized as a kind of rubber band. The power of instinct in general was its elasticity, an elasticity that sought forever to restore itself to its original shape—or, as he puts it, "an impulsion towards the restoration of a situation which once existed but was brought to an end by some external disturbance." He saw life, then, as the battlefield upon which the life and death instincts worked sometimes together, eventually apart.

Freud's theory of the death instinct is the most unpopular of all his constructions, more scorned even than the life-affirming theory of sexuality. The rejection of the theory of the death instinct is summed up in the argument of J. L. Grey: ". . . the fact that we all die is no proof that we purpose to die, any more than that we are all conceived is proof of a purpose in non-existence to become life."[94]

Freud himself offered the theory with some hesitation. "It remains to be seen," he said, "whether this construction will turn out to be serviceable. Although it arose from a desire to fix some of the most important theoretical ideas of psychoanalysis, it goes far beyond psychoanalysis." The conviction that we are all driven, over and beyond the exercise of our rational control, towards the dark and inevitable end does, of course, go far beyond psychoanalysis. It not only goes beyond it, but it negates in its implications the underlying thesis of Freud's whole discipline: that the unconscious forces to which we are subject can be tamed and put to social usefulness by the exercise of reason. We can only assume that as Freud entered the last two decades of his life he was preparing himself for death; that this preparation was reflected in his work; and that, although death took its time, possibly because of its partner's heroic will to survive, it nevertheless so pervaded his remaining years that he was willing to jeopardize the world he had evolved in defiance of it.

The books that came later, *The Future of an Illusion*, *Civilization and Its Discontents*, and *Moses and Monotheism*, leaped from the speculations which Freud adduced for the individual and applied them to society as a whole.

The Future of an Illusion deals with the "illusion" of religious feeling, and compares the effect of the consolations of religion, as Marx did, to a narcotic. It is written in the form of a running dialogue between the author and a hypothetical defender of the benefits of religion. The form is significant, for it represents not Freud and an opponent, but Freud and that part of his own nature which was as staunch an upholder of the faith as any churchman. To his opponent, who is finally forced to admit that perhaps religion is an illusion, but that man cannot do without its consolation, Freud makes answer: Certainly, man's life will be more difficult without. "He will be in the same position as the child who has left the home where he was so warm and comfortable. But, after all, is it not the destiny of childishness to be overcome? Man cannot remain a child forever; he must venture at last into the hostile world. This may be called 'education to reality'; need I tell you that it is the sole aim of my book to draw attention to the necessity for this advance?"[95]

For religion Freud wanted to substitute the primacy of the intelligence, the solutions of science. He answers his opponent's criticism of this point of view before the opponent has had a chance to voice it. "I know how difficult it is," he says, "to avoid illusions; perhaps even the hopes I have confessed to are of an illusory nature." But his illusions about science, he says, are not like the religious ones; they are not incapable of correction; they are not "delusional." Religion is like a childhood neurosis. On the other hand, he grants that his substitution of knowledge for religion may be inadequate, its application to the human race unjustified, and his optimism about its inspirational power without foundation.

But "we may insist as much as we like," Freud says, "that the human intellect is weak in comparison with human instincts, and be right in doing so. Nevertheless there is something peculiar about this weakness. The voice of the intellect is a soft one, but it does not rest until it has gained a hearing. Ultimately, after endlessly repeated rebuffs, it succeeds. This is one of the few points in which one may be optimistic about the future of mankind, but in itself it signifies not a little. And one can make it a starting-point for yet other hopes. The primacy of the intellect certainly lies in the far—far, but still probably not infinite—distance. And as it will presumably set itself the same aims that you expect to be realized by your God . . . we may say that our antagonism is only a temporary and not an irreconcilable one. . . . In the long run nothing can withstand reason and experience, and the contradiction religion offers to both is only too palpable. . . . We believe that it is possible for scientific work to discover something about the reality of the world through which we can increase our power and according to which we can regulate our life."[96]

"No," Freud concludes—and in doing so he reminds us

of the child who insists that he will sleep with his eyes open—"science is no illusion. But it would be an illusion to suppose that we could get anywhere else what it cannot give us." Thus, one of the world's most determined disillusionists falls into the trap of ruthlessly tearing from his life one of man's great "illusions," only to substitute for it another.

Throughout the pages of *The Future of an Illusion*, as in so many of Freud's works, there runs a personal statement disguised in general terms, a statement which in this case shows how the man of seventy arrived at his cold mountain peak of reason *ueber alles*. He says again—and this has now become a pervasive *leitmotif* of his work—that "for the individual, as for mankind in general, life is hard to endure. The culture in which he shares imposes on him some measure of privation, and other men occasion him a certain degree of suffering. . . . Man's seriously menaced self-esteem craves consolation, life and the universe must be rid of their terrors, and incidentally man's curiosity, reinforced, it is true, by the strongest practical motives, demands an answer."[97] He asserts that most men build their answer "out of the material offered by memories of the helplessness of their own childhood, and the childhood of the human race," and thus paint the picture of their God over the picture of their fathers. But this was not his way. He would not be dealt a truth that was acceptable to everyone else, and accept it for that reason. He says: "I was already a man of mature years when I stood for the first time on the hill of the Athenian Acropolis, between the temple ruins, looking out on to the blue sea. A feeling of astonishment mingled with my pleasure, which prompted me to say: then it really is true, what we used to be taught at school! How shallow and weak at that age must have been my belief in the real truth of what I heard if I can be so astonished to-day!"[98]

Some ten years later, in a paper called *A Disturbance of Memory at the Acropolis*, Freud confirmed the fact that his own rejection of authority and authoritative answers was bound up with his rejection of his father, no less than other men's acceptance of authority stems from their love of their fathers. He says in this paper: "To travel so far, to go so well on in life, seemed to me then beyond all possibilities. This was a consequence of the narrowness and poverty of our circumstances during my youth. . . . This has to do with the child's criticism of the father, with the undervaluation which took the place of the overvaluation of early childhood."

In *Civilization and Its Discontents,* published three years after *The Future of an Illusion,* Freud continued his study of man's battle against a restrictive, oppressive culture. The book is an attempt to trace genetically the course of man's search for happiness in a civilization which demands the renunciation of instinctual pleasure. Freud's analysis of the outcome of this search is not a happy one: "It is . . . the pleasure-principle which draws up the programme of life's programme. . . . [This principle] simply cannot be put into operation, the whole constitution of things runs counter to it; one might say the intention that man should be 'happy' is not in the scheme of 'Creation.'" What happens? Freud's answer is that "under the pressure of the various sources from which suffering comes, humanity tends to reduce its demands for happiness; the goal of the pleasure-principle is unattainable."

Civilization is made by men. Why, then, have they sown it with the seeds of discontent? There are a number of reasons, says Freud. First, love is opposed to culture. Second, love, or Eros, or libido, or the pleasure-principle, is characterized, like so many other physical forces, by inertia. It is disinclined to relinquish an old position in favour of a new one. Third—and this Freud considers to be the most important factor—man's aggressive inclinations, innate, independent and instinctual, form the most powerful obstacle to a more benign culture. He comes finally to the conclusion that the course of culture or civilization, like the course of individual man, is a struggle between Eros and Death.

Thus Freud applied the concept of the individual will to die to society as a whole. The sum of the parts, Freud came to believe, was no different from the individual whole. Man, nature, society—everything—hurled itself wilfully towards its own destruction; and the stormy aggressiveness he had seen so perfectly epitomized in the war was simply the external manifestation of this internal will. Self-avowed atheist though he was, the battle he envisaged between the forces of life and death was, in a sense, not very different from the church's conception of the struggle between Good and Evil. There was one difference: the faith which, for a man of religion, fights on the side of the Good fights without favour for a man of science on the side of Eros.

Although Freud had expressed his optimism about the eventual supremacy of reason in *The Future of an Illusion*, this optimism was apparently not strong enough to offset his conviction that the will to destroy must always be victorious over the will to live and create.

It is apparent from his private conversations at the time these books were published that this was the way he felt. He was approaching his seventy-fifth year, and the end of the first decade of his communion with the malignant cancerous growth of death. Although he told a visitor in 1930 that he still preferred "existence to extinction," he added: "Perhaps the Gods are kind to us by making life more disagreeable as we grow older. In the end, death seems less intolerable than the manifold burdens we carry." And, in the next breath: "Age with its manifest discomforts comes to all . . . the final victory always belongs to the conqueror worm. . . . I am perfectly content to know that the eternal nuisance of living will finally be done with."

He clung steadfastly to the uncomforting banners of reason, but he did for a brief period permit himself to look at a world whose existence he denied—the world of those people who are mystically convinced of a life after death. In 1919 he wrote a paper on *The "Uncanny,"* in 1922 one on *Dreams and Telepathy*, and in 1923 *A Neurosis of Demoniacal Possession in the Seventeenth Century*. None of these articles departed in any way from Freud's usual, rational approach. None of them admitted that there was any explanation other than rational of these "spirit" phenomena. But all of them contain suggestions that Freud's reasons for investigating the phenomena are not entirely impersonal. For example, he begins the paper on *The "Uncanny"* by saying that it has been a long time since he himself has known anything resembling an uncanny experience, and that he must translate himself into that state of feeling, and "awaken in himself the possibility of it" before he can write about it. Not so many pages later he contradicts himself in relating his experience on the street of "painted women" in the provincial Italian town. Of his experience, it will be recalled, he said, "a feeling overcame me, which I can only describe as uncanny." He is content, despite his lifelong predilection for analysing all such incidents down to the bare bone of the wish that inspired them, to ascribe his own and all other uncanny experiences to an inner involuntary "repetition compulsion."

In his strange paper on *Dreams and Telepathy* we find the same determination to reduce an extra-rational phenomenon to a rational basis. This time, telepathic experiences are traced back to emotions belonging to the sphere of the Œdipus complex. Again, the paper begins with a disclaimer and winds up with a virtual affirmation. "You will know," he says, "that the connection between dreams and telepathy is commonly held to be a very intimate one; I shall propound the view that the two have little to do with each other, and that if the existence of telepathic dreams were established there would be no need to alter our conception of dreams in any way." He proceeds then to demolish a few so-called telepathic dreams which have come to his attention. But in the doing there again creeps into the carefully analytic passages the suggestion that for all the explaining there remains something out of the field of vision of his omniscient seer's eye.

When psychoanalysis and occultism encounter each other, he says, psychoanalysis has "all our instinctive prepossessions against it"; and occultism "is met half-way by powerful and mysterious sympathies. I am not, however, going to take up the position that I am nothing but a psychoanalyst, that the problems of occultism do not concern me: you would rightly judge that to be only an evasion of the problem. On the contrary, I maintain that it would be a great satisfaction to me if I could convince myself and others, on unimpeachable evidence, of the existence of telepathic processes. . . ." There speaks the wish for satisfaction which undoubtedly motivated the paper. At the end he says: "There remains one element of the apparently intimate connection between telepathy and dreams which is not affected by any of these considerations: namely, the incontestable fact that sleep creates favourable conditions for telepathy." In other words, the existence of telepathy, which was questioned in the introduction to the paper, is now tacitly admitted. He proceeds: "We must add, however, that no one has a right to take exception to telepathic occurrences on the ground that the event and the presentiment . . . do not exactly coincide in astronomical time. . . . If the phenomenon of telepathy is only an activity of the unconscious mind, then no fresh problem lies before us. The laws of unconscious mental life may then be taken for granted as applying to telepathy."[99]

He is aware that these remarks add up to an apparent admission of the existence of telepathy. But he hastens, away from the forbidden fruits of the world that stretches beyond rational control, to retract that admission. "Have I given you the impression," he asks, "that I am secretly inclined to support the reality of telepathy in the occult sense? If so, I should very much regret that it is so difficult to avoid giving such an impression. In reality, however, I was anxious to be strictly impartial. I have every reason to be so, for I have no opinion; I know nothing about it."

The paper on demoniacal possession is significant in that it reflects Freud's preoccupation with death. It is not startling that he chose to investigate at this time a medieval counterpart who felt that he had entered into a compact with the Devil and was thus possessed by an evil destructive spirit who demanded his death in exchange for granting him a few easier years of life.

These three papers present cumulative evidence of Freud's die-hard absolutism. In the face of an inclination which led him, as it leads all men, to try to understand those things which loom beyond the sphere of our rational control, he brought the will not to understand.* Straight into the infinitely frightening face of impending death, a death he had convinced himself he was responsible for, Freud hurled his defiance of comfort: Come if you must! But I insist on saying I do not believe that the land you inhabit is a real one. Look, I can destroy it with the blowtorch I have invented to puncture the real world. You cannot communicate with the living through telepathy, or occultism. You cannot enter into the spirit of man with pacts signed in blood. I am still the strong man I convinced myself I was from childhood on. I will look you in the face without hope, without comfort, without faith.

Is is only, as we have seen, in the reverberations of this shout of defiance that the whisper of a plaintive, ashamed, apologetic question emerges. The question: "Or will I?"

* The unconscious, that irrational domain which for all time will be associated with Freud's name, is, of course, a different kettle of fish. For Freud felt that the power of the unconscious was harnessable; that it was, in other words, eminently suited for rational control.

15

The Larger World of Psychoanalysis

The first World War opened the eyes of official medicine to the value of the psychoanalytic idea. While the medical profession still was careful to keep its distance, it came at last, through the observation of war neuroses, to a recognition of the significance of psychic factors in producing neurotic disturbances. Some of the psychoanalytic conceptions, such as "the advantage of being ill" and the "flight into illness," suddenly became popular. By the end of the war it was evident even to medical die-hards that "shell-shock," so-called, was not necessarily caused by physical concussion, and that the many cases of hysterical paralysis of strategic organs, like arms, legs, and trigger fingers, were rooted not so much in the conscious desire to malinger as in the unconscious mechanisms which Freud first described. The last psychoanalytic congress before the German collapse, which was held at Budapest in 1918, was attended by official representatives of the allied governments of the Central European powers, and they agreed to the establishment of psychoanalytic stations for the treatment of war neuroses. Although the war ended before this could be put into effect, a psychoanalytic institute and clinic for veterans was established in Berlin in 1920, and Ferenczi, during the Bolshevist rule in Hungary, conducted a successful course of psychoanalytic instruction at the University of Budapest.

While the great majority of doctors and psychiatrists were still either hesitant or hostile to psychoanalysis, a number of scientists of high standing and of famous men of letters treated it with increasing respect. Most significantly, and, to Freud's mind, most regrettably—that part of the post-war world represented by the *avant-garde* intellectuals and their hangers-on among the rich and frivolous began to seize upon psychoanalysis and the most convenient of its tenets as a philosophical justification for sexual license. Among these sensation-seekers, psychoanalysis became a fad.

In America, people like Mabel Dodge, "whose spirit . . . like a bird within a glass-walled room . . . was desperately beating its wings against the impediments between it and freedom," had found psychoanalysis during the war years; they approached it, as they had Buddhism, Christian Science, the cult of Gertrude Stein, anarchy, and collections of old glass, with an intense and jumpy need for faith and purpose. Mabel Dodge began to be psychoanalysed by Dr. Smith Ely Jelliffe, one of the leading psychoanalysts in America. At first she loved it. She enjoyed Jelliffe's "amusing intuition." She said: "It became an absorbing game to play with oneself, reading one's motives, and trying to understand the symbols by which the soul expressed itself. Psychoanalysis was apparently a kind of tattle-taling. . . . I longed to draw others into the new world where I found myself: a world where things fitted into a set of definitions and terms that I had never even dreamt of. It simplified all problems to name them. There was the Electra complex, and the Œdipus complex, and there was the Libido with its manifold activities, seeking every chance for outlet, and then all that thing about Power and Money!"

She did not find this entertaining tattle-taling "at all dangerous. It was interesting," she said, "to watch my soul provide exciting subjects to discuss with Jelliffe. Whenever things got dull, something would turn up from down below to keep the ball rolling—and he and I chased it about.

He told me more strange and fascinating oddities and now I have forgotten them nearly all!"[100]

Mabel Dodge's judgments could never be considered typical, but they were symptomatic of the lay attitude towards psychoanalysis in America during the war and post-war period. The serious and informed were outnumbered by the enthusiasts like Mabel Dodge. What these enthusiasts lacked in depth of understanding they made up in the loudness of their hallelujahs. Freud, who saw psychoanalysis spreading slowly but pervasively throughout Europe, was appalled by the enthusiasm of the American response, for he felt it to be superficial and uncritical. His original prejudice against America was reinforced. When, in his writing, he needed to epitomize shallowness, he would automatically think of America. He wrote in *Thoughts on War and Death,* in talking about life that is lived without depth: "It becomes as flat, as superficial, as one of those American flirtations in which it is from the first understood that nothing is to happen, contrasted with a continental love affair in which both partners must constantly bear in mind the serious consequences." To a friend, in the late 1920s, he said: "Americans are clever generalizers. They are rarely creative thinkers." This uncomplimentary opinion of America he maintained until the day of his death; to Sachs, who had by that time moved to America, he said, shortly before he died: "I know that I have at least *one* friend in America."

Afraid no less of the manner in which he was being accepted than of the manner in which he had been rejected. Freud did a characteristic thing. He bound to himself, with a gift of identical Græco-Roman intaglio rings similar to one he himself always wore, the six most loyal disciples in whom he placed the most trust: Karl Abraham, Max Eitingon, Ferenczi, Ernest Jones, Otto Rank and Sachs. The rings, as Sachs says, "had a certain symbolic significance." They made these six men feel that they belonged to a group within a group, whose centre of gravity was Freud. Nor did Freud allow the recognition of the gift's significance to remain implicit. At the first psychoanalytic congress held after the war at The Hague in 1920, he called the six men together and unfolded a plan to them.

Henceforward they, with him, were to form a co-ordinated but strictly anonymous group. The duty of this cabal, like the duty of the Marxian vanguard of the proletariat, would be to direct the expanding psychoanalytic movement according to predetermined plan. The future of psychoanalysis must not be left to chance, he said, nor allowed to founder on the rocks of factionalism or personal ambition. To protect it, the men of the seven rings must work in secret, and apart from other members of the psychoanalytic brotherhood. They were, since they lived in different places—Freud and Rank in Vienna, Abraham, Eitingon and Sachs in Berlin, Ferenczi in Budapest and Jones in London—to supervise the affairs of psychoanalysis in their various countries. They were to correspond with each other at regular intervals, and the letters were to be passed around to every member of the group so that all could be kept up to date on events on each front. The agenda of these letters, Freud instructed them, were to include: reports of local organizational activities; "questions, comments, advice, discussion designed to clarify the current problems and to trace a general line for our policy," as Sachs recalls; and finally, matters of personal interest, whether they were scientific projects or grievances. After each psychoanalytic congress, the seven men were to meet for a few days for personal discussion and communion. If extraordinary occasions arose, they were to meet between conventions, which were held biennially.

Between 1920 and 1925, the years of greatest peace and steady progress in the psychoanalytic movement, this plan was carried out. Work in the various psychoanalytic institutes for which these men were responsible developed smoothly; new and talented workers were attracted to the psychoanalytic vineyard, and were trained by the seven men. But peace and the symbolic tie of mystic union did not last long. Rank published his book attributing all neurotic symptoms and much of the world's trouble to the trauma of birth, without consulting his six confrères. This was interpreted by five members of the group as heresy, *lèse-majesté* and nonsense. Ferenczi was more or less on Rank's side. Although Freud tried for a while to arbitrate the differences, this was the time of his first, incomplete operation, and death seemed imminent. Then Rank moved to Paris, which was not particularly sympathetic to any brand of psychoanalysis, and shortly thereafter Abraham, whose work in Berlin had been outstanding, died. Sachs, Jones and Freud tried to keep the cabal alive, but its vitality began to diminish.

Thus, until cancer attacked him, Freud kept a tight check-rein on the organizational affairs of psychoanalysis. After that, for the sixteen remaining years of his life, his hold on the scientific and secular development of psychoanalysis grew imperceptibly slacker. Despite the fact that the majority of psychoanalysts clung rigidly to the letter of the Freudian lore, new developments occurred and new theories were propounded which attested to the vitality of the movement, as distinct from that of its founder.

The psychoanalysts of the early 1920s had assimilated Freud's basic concepts, but they were prone to jump directly from surface symptoms and associations to deep interpretation in terms of historic infantile situations, which the patient was far from ready to accept. Eventual dissatisfaction and frustration among the analysts led to a search for new therapeutic answers, beginning in the late twenties. The new answers of the second period of psychoanalysis' development again borrowed from Freud, as Jung and Adler had done, and made one of his concepts the cornerstone of a "new" theory. Early among these attempts to hack a path out of the maze of therapeutic frustration was Otto Rank's system of "transference analysis." Freud had already said that the working out of transference—the emotional relationship of the patient to the analyst—was basic to the therapeutic situation. Rank now made it the only factor in the therapeutic situation. Self-knowledge did not have to be based on a knowledge of unconscious mechanisms. It was enough, Rank said, if the analytic situation taught the patient the facts of a good relationship with another person. In the knowledge of such a relationship, the patient would discover his own self in all its uniqueness.

Other schools of analytic thought took opposite paths from Rank's. Karl Abraham decided that the more remote from consciousness an impulse was, and the earlier the period to which a traumatic incident or a fantasy could be traced, the more valuable a signpost it was to an understanding of the patient's neurosis. He attempted, with Teutonic orderliness, to find the precise historical point at which every neurotic symptom had become fixed.

Precise as was Abraham's approach, the British school of psychoanalysis, led by Ernest Jones and Melanie Klein, went further. Freud had implied that the neurosis of a grown man was constructed in diseased fashion from the wounds of a childhood neurosis, mainly in the years from three to six. Jones and Klein suggested that these three years were not the conditioning ones: what counted was the first year of life, the "prehistoric," absolutely primitive condition of man before the power of reason had much of a chance to exert itself. From this perspective Freud's conclusions in terms of the later emotional conflicts of childhood, such as penis-envy and the fear of castration, appeared not so much erroneous as superficial—the scabs upon the sores of deeper unconscious hurts.

Abraham, Jones and Klein did not quarrel with Freud. They simply penetrated deeper into one aspect of his conceptual construction. Analysts who chose another path of deviation from Freud, those who are now headed by Karen Horney, believe, despite the lip service paid by their leader to the ground-work established by Freud, that they are engaged in a holy, albeit sociological, crusade against Freud's predominantly biologic bias. Their battle cry is "Environment!" not "Heredity!" They believe that modern man's neuroses are produced not so much by the faulty functioning of instinctual drives as by cultural influences: our times, disturbed human relationships, the conflicts inherent in a Christian-capitalist society. They hold, in opposition to Freud's theory, that disturbed sexuality is not the cause of neurosis, but its frequent outcome. Neurotic development, they say, is the result of disturbed human relationships. Because this school minimizes the importance of instinctual drives, among them the aggressiveness and death impulse Freud set so much store by, they are proud of proclaiming their "optimism" and contrasting it with Freud's "pessimism." They do not in truth share Freud's profoundly pessimistic view of human nature and his consequent doubts about the efficacy of psychoanalysis in cutting a swathe through the jungle of human misery. Where Freud spoke with the voice of the prophet predicting doom, they speak in cheery, extroverted tones predicting eventual victory.

The therapy of the Horney school owes more to Adler than it does to Freud. Emphasis is more on the analysis of the patient's ego than of his unconscious. Far more study is devoted to the patient's current life, his rivalries, his insecurities, his surface conflicts and his human relationships than to an investigation of his childhood. Horneyites do, however, use the technique of free association and the transference situation in much the same way as Freud. Some members of the Horney school believe that a patient who has successfully concluded one of their analyses emerges with a blueprint of his whole future life legibly spread out before him. They confidently expect that this completely whole, soundly integrated, perfect round of a cured neurotic will function with oiled precision in a world which is still bent on making him as sick as he was in the first place.* It is more than likely that their expectation, in the light of the surface nature of a Horneyite analysis, is illusory.

A third school of psychoanalysis, approaching the proportions of a cult, is that formed by Wilhelm Reich—expelled from the International Psychoanalytic Society in 1933—and his adherents. Unlike the Horneyites, who minimize the importance of sexuality, the Reichites go even further than Freud in believing that sex is everything. Briefly, Reich says that our whole modern society is sick primarily because it is sexually starved. It is the quality of this sexual starvation that is so appalling, and the quality

* These are the beliefs of some of Dr. Horney's followers, not of herself.

centres in the condition of the orgasm, to whose study Reich devoted a book, *The Function of the Orgasm,* the Bible of the Reich school. The thesis of the book is that all physical, mental and social ailments, from ulcers to Fascism, stem from "orgiastic impotence," which is not the inability to attain an orgasm, but the inability to derive sufficient pleasure from it. This inability, which according to Reich is virtually universal, stems mainly from "the patriarchal family," and its "compulsive morality." All the social and political ailments of the modern world are simply large-scale projections of the unhappy sex-starved condition of the individual.

How one discovers whether he belongs to the orgiastically potent who shall inherit the earth, or to the orgiastically impotent who are doomed to swim around sullenly in the sinkhole of the modern world as it is, is left chiefly to subjective determination. There are certain infallible indicators, according to Reich, of whether you belong with the élite. First, if your ability to derive the fullest possible measure of high-quality sexual satisfaction is complete, you will be set apart from the sewer-dwellers by your high colour, moist and elastic skin, and the full-blooded healthiness of your genitals—in brief, by your enormous vitality and well being. Second, this vitality will be reflected in your enormous power for creative work. Finally, this unleashed creative energy will not allow you to cling to a dull mechanical job. No assembly line or file cabinet can hold the orgiastically potent and smother him into neurotic submission. His is the world of artistic creation—such a Reichite world as already blossoms in fact near Carmel in California, where a young, blue-jeaned, orgiastically potent intelligentsia produces incomprehensible poetry, ceramics, and bits of broken glass strung on wire, between bouts of proving their orgiastic right to this world.

Meanwhile, between the extreme biologic and extreme cultural poles of psychoanalytic development, the psychoanalysts who adhere more closely to the precepts laid down by Freud, and who form the great majority of practising analysts, pursue their way. There are among them the extreme orthodox, who will move not a jot nor a tittle away from the law as it was handed down on the Berggasse. These are the men who have inherited the psychological attitude that had a basis of reality when it was born in Freud, the attitude of suspicion and hostility evoked by a suspicious and hostile world in the infancy of psychoanalysis. Fortunately for the future of psychoanalysis, these sterile propagators of the faith do not wield the influence of those who feel free to experiment within the Freudian framework with both the theory and practice of psychoanalysis.

Into this Freudian but expansionist group falls the work of Anna Freud and others similarly minded. They believe that Freud's great emphasis on the importance of the instinctual drives must be brought into better balance and integrated with a more rounded psychology of the ego. This sounds like Horney's thesis, but the difference is that they study the ego not only in its relation to the outside world, but equally in its relation to the inner world of instinctual drives; and primary emphasis is laid on the interrelation between the two. In her study of defense mechanisms, Anna Freud was concerned with this thesis. And she demonstrated that man uses similar techniques in dealing with the world of outer reality and with the inner reality of his instinctual drives and anxieties.

This Freudian school is concerned with minutiae—with a diamond faceted analysis of each phase of human personality in terms of both its conscious and unconscious elements. It frowns on the short-circuit interpretations that characterized the analysts of the 1920s, and instead inches downward and backward with the tenacity of an earthworm, towards the broadest possible, detailed view of the neurotic career.

Franz Alexander, one of Freud's most gifted and most ambitious disciples, who now heads the Chicago Psychoanalytic Institute, is currently spearheading another Freudian revisionist movement, which is known in some quarters as the "neo-Freudian" school. Alexander, like many Freudian psychoanalysts practising to-day, sensibly holds that the spirit of Freud's teachings is unexceptionable, but that many of his specific notions, such as the theory of the libido, are highly untenable and primitive in orientation. He and his followers point out with justice that the theoretical formulations of psychoanalysis have not kept pace with our rapidly expanding view of human personality—a view which includes, as Horney has over-emphasized, all the environmental and cultural forces which condition personality. He is heartily in favour of a total understanding of the human personality as opposed to a rigid adherence to theoretical abstractions, no matter how brilliantly fathered.

These beliefs have led not to a new, but to a more substantially founded attempt to overhaul and reform the cumbersome therapeutic technique. Other analysts who have attempted a short cut through the lengthy therapeutic process have usually overemphasized the significance of one part of the technique at the expense of other parts. Thus, some analysts have insisted that emotional working out of the conflicts is sufficient; others that intellectual insight more than anything else is the answer; and another group that the heart of the cure lies in the gradual removal of the amnesia that surrounds infantile memories. None of these innovations which isolated single aspects of the therapeutic technique ever gained wide acceptance, although they were all devised in the interests of a shorter therapy. The kind of therapy practised by Alexander and his co-workers at the Chicago Institute of Psychoanalysis, however, is becoming more and more widespread in practice, and is used not only by the Chicago Institute, but increasingly by analysts all over the country.

This form of treatment, which is still evolving, is distinguished by two newly emphasized factors: First, in lieu of the traditional Freudian attitude of allowing the treatment to take its own course, with the watching analyst functioning in a more or less passive manner, this school stresses the value of a plan of treatment. In other words, after appraising the patient's personality and problems, the analyst decides in advance whether he needs a supportive or more penetrating type of treatment, or whether the job is mainly a question of changing the external conditions of his life. Second, they recommend the conscious use of various techniques employed in a flexible manner, with tactics shifted to fit the needs of the moment. Among the modifications of the standard technique entailed by the emphasis on flexibility are: interviews of a more direct character than the sessions of free association—which are also used; changing the frequency of the interviews, depending on the needs of the moment; advising the patient directly about problems in his daily life; making use of long or short interruptions in preparation for ending the treatment; directing the transference relationship, instead of letting it run its natural course, in order to meet the specific needs of the case—and so on.

None of these modifications is in itself "new." All, Alexander says, have been used on occasion by a large number of psychoanalysts as more or less accidental or "practical" measures. But the contribution of the analysts who, like Alexander, believe in this shorter, more directed route of psychoanalysis, is that they have systematized and clarified the use of these modifications and are working towards integrating them into the standard procedure of analytic therapy.

Other procedures based on psychoanalytic techniques have emerged from their wartime use in the treatment of psychoneuroses among the armed forces. Although these methods are relatively untried, and may eventually be found to effect only a superficial cure, they are valuable in indicating a more widespread use of psychoanalytic techniques in the treatment of mental ailments. Among them is the use of narcosynthesis. In this procedure, the patient is given a dose of a sedative like sodium pentothal which decreases the intensity of his immediate symptoms. Under its influence he is induced by an analyst to talk and tell what is bothering him. He usually not only talks, but emotionally relives the traumatic situations which have caused his neurosis. The analyst then fortifies this relief on an unconscious level with talks conducted while the patient is no longer under the influence of the drug.

There are other methods and other approaches developing in psychoanalytic therapy. But these will serve to indicate the wide experimentation that is being pursued. It is apparent that psychoanalysis as a theory and a practice is a vital, evolving body of knowledge on the road towards resolution and further development in the hands of the synthesizers of the divergent viewpoints.

With the rise of the Nazis and the disappearance of Vienna as the seat of psychoanalysis, America became the asylum for the psychoanalytic refugees. Freud's pupils, dislodged by the Nazis from their institutes and debarred from practice, emigrated, with few exceptions, to America. Here the largest psychoanalytic institutes were organized, the great profusion of books and articles were published, conservative psychiatric circles were most deeply influenced, and the hottest factional psychoanalytic battles were waged. Despite Freud's suspicion of the popularity his theories enjoyed in America, despite his scorn for America's ways and manners, history perpetrated another of those paradoxes which marked Freud's life: America became in the late 'thirties, and continues now to be, the psychoanalytic seat from which most major developments stem.

Now, with the war ended and with the spirit of strife, dissension and dissection giving way to a new synthesizing, less polemic approach, "the American era of psychoanalysis" is on the road towards a more fruitful result. Psychoanalysis, in its first American phase, centred around the eastern seaboard. Now the movement has seeped westward, and great psychoanalytic centres, born in the thirties, are spearheading the expansionist movement. Affiliated and related with the Chicago Institute in Chicago, which has already accomplished outstanding psychoanalytic research work, is the group centred in Los Angeles around Dr. Ernst Simmel, an old friend and disciple of Freud's. In Topeka, Kansas, the Menninger Clinic is also doing notable experimental and research work in psychoanalysis.

By the early 1930s the psychoanalytic approach to human problems had tinctured the thinking of the world. Whether people completely understood what they were saying or not, Freudian terms such as "complex," "libido," "sublimation" and "fixation" had crept into their everyday language. In the twenties, awareness of Freud and his discoveries had been limited to the *avant-garde* and to the so-called intelligentsia. By the next decade the Freudian word had seeped down to pulp magazines, comic strips, musical comedies and advertising copy. Learned journals and technical articles designed for scientists referred to his doctrines. The greatest of his contemporaries began to seek him out—Einstein, Thomas Mann and Romain Rolland among them. His birthdays, which had passed uncelebrated by the world, began with his seventieth to be occasions for world-wide acclamation. In 1926 Vienna, which had never seen fit to accord him full academic recognition, granted him the freedom of the city.

His seventy-fifth birthday was celebrated not only in Vienna but in London and New York as well, and congratulatory messages poured in on him from all over the world. Orchids, of which Freud was particularly fond, arrived to fill his wife's modest conservatory. The Vienna Medical Society, the same august group which had laughed derisively at his first exposition of psychoanalysis, made him an honorary member. A tablet was unveiled marking his birthplace at Freiberg, and ceremonies were held there honouring him and his work. On this occasion Dr. Julius Wagner-Jauregg, the Viennese psychiatrist who had epitomized the opposition of the medical world to Freud, arose to say: "Recognition by enemies is worth more than any amount of praise from supporters."

Freud received the acclaim with the same weary resignation with which he had received the rejection. He attended none of the celebrations, accepted none of the honours in person, and delegated Anna to act for him. Even the relatives who had formerly celebrated his birthdays with him were not permitted to see him. Suffering, withdrawn, and unmoved by the honours which he had wished for all his life and which now came too late, he was off in the Austrian Alps. Eight months before this birthday celebration his mother had died at the age of ninety-three. Like her son, she had been hearty and extraordinarily energetic in her old age. But unlike him, she had been cheerful until shortly before her death. On the evening before his seventieth birthday Freud had gone to visit her to receive her congratulations, in order to spare her the long trip to his house from the suburb in which she lived. The next morning, the first visitor to ring his doorbell was his mother. Her ninetieth birthday had been the occasion for a celebration by Ischl, the Austrian summer resort she had visited regularly for thirty years. She was serenaded by the town band, and presented with the freedom of the town. And she received a constant stream of visitors bearing gifts and congratulations all day. In the evening her granddaughter remarked solicitously, "You must be terribly tired, granny." "Why?" the surprised matriarch demanded. "I haven't done a stroke of work all day."

Freud's eightieth birthday, in 1936, was again the occasion for public and private celebration. Articles commemorating the event appeared in dozens of languages. In most of them Freud's work was praised. An address was presented to him by many of the outstanding men of his time—scientists, scholars, authors, artists. On this festive occasion, as on the others, Freud kept himself in seclusion. He appeared at none of the ceremonies, and no one was admitted to congratulate him except his family and closest friends. He explained his withdrawal by saying that his work was done, that he owed the world no more public appearances. What he wrote in the latter part of his life, he said, "could have been eliminated without loss. It could also have been produced by others. I wrote with an open heart and received little thanks. I cannot recommend my manner of life or activity to anyone else." He did, however, despite his lack-lustre view of the festivities, allow himself one pleasure: Thomas Mann came quietly to read only to Freud and his family the paper he had presented at the public meeting in his honour.

For all Freud's lack of regard for his manner of life and "activity," the world by this time thought otherwise. Whether or not people agreed with Freud's concept of the Œdipus complex, they were prone to trace their current difficulties back to their childhood situations. Whether they preferred the age of innocence to the era of infantile sexuality, Freud's doctrines had so far revolutionized the field of child psychology that they were beginning to rear their children in a spirit diametrically opposed to the rigid authority which characterized Freud's own childhood. Where their sex life had been a subject neither for conscious consideration nor discussion, where it had been blanketed under centuries of traditionally imposed reticence and guilt, people were emerging from an era of sexual license (which had been their first understanding of what Freud was saying) into a more sane, more balanced recognition of their fundamental natures.

These attitudes and these points of view came to them not from a study of Freud's work but indirectly, through novels, plays, magazines and newspapers. Revolutionary as Freud's concepts proved to be in the field of normal and abnormal psychology, his influence in the arts was greater. And of all artists the writer, because his preoccupation, like Freud's, is with men's motivation, was most influenced by Freudian concepts. Whether it be the novel or poetry, drama or biography, historical literature or surrealist outpourings, detective fiction or movie scripts which are examined, there is apparent, not only in the content but increasingly in the form, an overwhelming concern with those unconscious emotional forces in human behaviour and society which Freud first charted for his era.

Art and literature, which had been primarily concerned with a depiction of the surface world of reality, began to penetrate below the surface in order to expose the hidden motives and drives which Freud had uncovered. The workings of the unconscious mind began to take precedence, as a matter of concern to artists, over the description of the conscious mind. For many writers and artists the psychoanalytic revelation was, as Thomas Mann said it was for him, "a revolutionary force." "With it," he says, "a blithe scepticism has come into the world, a mistrust which unmasks all the schemes and subterfuges of our own souls. Once roused and on the alert, it cannot be put to sleep again. It infiltrates life, undermines its raw naïveté, takes from it the strain of its own ignorance. . . ." The impact of Freud's way of thinking was so pervasive that more than one critic has called our literary era "the Freudian epoch."

This epoch began in America when the intellectuals and artists reached such a state of psychoanalytic fervour that they would rather "psych" each other, as they called it, than eat. Although Walter Lippmann had in *A Preface to Morals*, published in 1914, shown a substantial and serious understanding of the Freudian doctrine, the Bohemians of the twenties, whose main intellectual concern was psychoanalysis, went off on a more naïve track, which was reflected in their work. Floyd Dell, for example, who soon became one of the leading apostles of the movement, and who quickly achieved wide popularity with novels like *Moon Calf*, began to be analyzed in 1916 "not for any particular neurotic difficulty," he said, "but because I thought it might be helpful to me in my love life and literary work." Dell helped Max Eastman edit *The Masses*, which adopted Freud as a colleague in spirit and used him as a springboard from which to stump for greater freedom in sex relations, more liberal divorce laws, woman's suffrage, and a general reevaluation of social and moral restrictions.

Among the radicals who spoke for the post-war intellectual revolt, Freud provided inexhaustible food for thought. But they gulped him in haste, and digested him poorly. American fiction of the twenties reflected the resultant psychoanalytic dyspepsia. Novels by Waldo Frank, Sherwood Anderson, F. Scott Fitzgerald and Ben Hecht were concerned with various aspects of sex, which, if they were not directly inspired by psychoanalysis, at least reflected the preoccupation of the era with the open discussion of sex which had been set in motion by Freud. Sherwood Anderson wrote in *Dark Laughter*: "If there is anything you do not understand in human life, consult the works of Dr. Freud." Frank, Anderson, and with them novelists like Conrad Aiken, Dreiser and Ludwig Lewisohn were also more seriously imbued with the Freudian spirit.

Dreiser said of Freud: "I shall never forget my first encounter with his *Three Contributions to a Theory of Sex*, his *Totem and Taboo*, and his *Interpretation of Dreams*. At that time, and even now, every paragraph came as a revelation to me—a strong, revealing light thrown on some of the darkest problems that haunted and troubled me and my work. And reading him has helped me in my studies of life and man. I said at that time, and I repeat now, that he reminded me of a conqueror who has taken a city, entered its age-old, hoary prisons and there generously proceeded to release from their gloomy and rusted cells the prisoners of formulae, faiths and illusions which have racked and worn man for hundreds and thousands of years. The light that he has thrown on the human mind! Its vagaries and destructive delusions and their cure! It is to me at once colossal and beautiful!"[101]

The twenties were in any case a time of self-examination, and psychoanalysis helped to turn writers' eyes inward. All of these men produced novels of introspection which bear the hallmarks of the analytic viewpoint. Their subject matter was the psychological implications and antecedents of human emotions and reactions. In their novels psychoanalytic doctrines are employed often with no great subtlety, but sometimes with great effectiveness.

These more important American writers of the twenties drew upon psychoanalysis seriously, if naïvely, in their work. Other writers of the era were content to make their obeisance to Freud by satirizing him. Rose Macaulay's *Dangerous Age*, published in New York in 1921, dealt wittily with psychoanalysis as an answer to a foolish and lonely old lady's need to talk to someone about herself. Rose Macaulay's old lady liked her analyst far better than her priest. Such grotesque conceptions of what psychoanalysis meant to the popular mind were also dealt with by Aldous Huxley in *Antic Hay;* by Susan Glaspell in an early play, *Suppressed Desires*, put on by the Provincetown Players; by such observers of cultural phenomena as Simeon Strunsky, who in 1919 wrote an article, "The Scandal of Euclid: A Freudian Analysis," which reviewed a hypothetical book called "Sex Elements in the First Five Books of Euclid." In it he traced Euclid's preoccupation with the "eternal triangle" to "a profound attachment developed by the geometer at the age of two for his grandmother on the father's side."

Although the decade of the 1930's was moved by the need for physical, material answers more than individual solutions, Freud and the way he had pointed were not lost sight of. The debate raged: was it possible to pay allegiance to the standard-bearers of the two decades—were the doctrines of Freud and Marx mutually exclusive or complementary? A few saw nothing irreconcilable in the two bodies of theory. But, for the most part, Marxists were scornful of the answers of psychoanalysis, professing to see in it, at its best, only the possibility of a successful adjustment to a sick society. Besides, psychoanalysis was for the rich. In a nation which could not spare a dime, the chance for the psychoanalyst to prove his merit was slight.

The old controversies with the Church and the Press, with the powers of outraged morality, were held over for continuous performance in another decade. Throughout the twenties Freud was attacked by churchmen on the grounds that he had pre-empted their domain of the confessional, their Devil, their doctrine of original sin—to all of which ancient properties of the Church he had affixed new labels. Freud was regarded by churchmen as an atheistic barbarian invader of the holy territory which stretched clearly defined between the boundaries of Good and Evil. Greater even than his sin of trespassing into this territory was the fact that he offered his unfortunate communicants neither a set of moral standards nor an absolution bathed in divine grace. And now, in the thirties, a new note was added to the outcry against Freud's emphasis on sex. The new critics said that psychoanalysis gave us nothing to substitute for its agitation against religious ethics and moral inhibitions. Articles called "The Danger of Psychoanalysis," "The Failure of Psychoanalysis," "The Treatment of Psychoanalysis," "The Freudian Illusion," peppered the pages of popular magazine and scholarly quarterly alike. In the middle thirties a new psychological enthusiasm arose briefly to threaten Freud's hegemony—John B. Watson's school of Behaviourism. And in 1938 a French publication compared Freud to Hitler.

They were alike, the author maintained, in their romantic preoccupation with the irrational sources of behaviour.

Most of this criticism sustained and continued the attacks made on Freudianism in the twenties. But throughout it, and played almost backstage against the central drama of Marxism, there began to emerge indications of a sounder understanding and a better evaluation of Freud and his place in modern thought. This understanding became evident in the literary output of the writers of the 1930's, though it is doubtful whether more than a handful of the many writers who were influenced by Freud's doctrines actually read very much of Freud. But the advantage which psychoanalysis enjoyed over other bodies of theory for the artistic mind none the less made it inevitable that Freud should wield a strong influence over creative writing. The fact that psychoanalysis shed a new light on the study of character and human behaviour, and so led the artist towards new perspectives and new viewpoints, explains in part its grip on the imagination of the artist. Equally significant is the fact that psychoanalysis gave the artist himself new clues towards the problem of his own behaviour, and so provided him with a newly equipped laboratory for the creation of his fictional characters.

But the artist is himself, by reason of his creative ability, an independent student of human nature. The conclusions he draws from his own direct experience often have little to do with the theoretical knowledge he has gained. Thus, it would be unreasonable to assume that Freud's influence on writing was directly a dominant one. Indirectly, his influence has been enormous.

James Joyce, whose *Ulysses* and *Finnegans Wake* are generally considered to be quintessential products of the psychoanalytic school of writing, was as much motivated in his exploration of various states of consciousness, in his use of dreams, dream symbols, and the language which arises from free association, by his own personal inclinations as he was by any familiarity with psychoanalysis. It is true that Joyce was exposed to psychoanalysis, first casually in Trieste, and later intensively in Zürich, where he lived during the most fruitful years of its development under Jung. In the isolation of Zürich, where Jung's and Freud's theories were the boldest, newest intellectual stimulus, he could hardly have been unaware of psychoanalysis. Nevertheless, when Mrs. Harold McCormick, Rockefeller's daughter, the axis around whom the Zürich psychoanalytic group revolved, contributed a thousand francs towards Joyce's support on the condition that he be psychoanalysed, he refused.

By 1922, however, Joyce had read almost all of Freud's work, and much of Jung's. And, as *Ulysses* and *Finnegans Wake* show, his understanding of psychoanalysis was far from superficial. This understanding contributes to his penetrating exploration of the unconscious minds of his characters. And, as Frederick J. Hoffman has pointed out,* "his conception of character motivation recognizes all of the bases for human relationship which psychoanalysis has identified." Joyce made use of the analytic idea in the same way in which he made use of other emotional and intellectual stimuli which were part of his experience. Psychoanalytic truths in Joyce's novels are not, as they were in the novels of Ludwig Lewisohn for example, the denuded clinical facts of the psychoanalytic couch. They are the integrated product of an imagination which has transmuted them from cold science into rich art. Joyce is no "Freudian" writer, but he belongs definitely to the "Freudian epoch."

Of D. H. Lawrence, another writer with great psychoanalytic perception, much the same thing can be said. Lawrence's *leit-motif* is Freud's *leit-motif*: man is a sexual animal, and the power of sex is the strength of his wellbeing. Lawrence was also preoccupied with the problems which psychoanalysis brought to the attention of the world—the problems of incest horror, and the Œdipus situation. But *Sons and Lovers,* which was published in 1913, and which psychoanalysts called the most penetrating study of the Œdipus complex in English literature, was written before Lawrence had more than a nodding ac-

* In *Freudianism and the Literary Mind.*

quaintance with Freud. Later, to be sure, when he met Frieda, who became his wife, he became interested in Freud and not only read him in the original but consulted over the course of a long period with Dr. Max Eder, a psychoanalyst who had long been associated with Freud. But he was soon disappointed with what he called psychoanalysis' "odour of the laboratory." He disliked its predilection for picking over feelings, and complained that psychoanalysts "can only help you more completely *to make your own feelings*. They can never let you *have* any real feelings." And he wrote to his friend Mabel Dodge, that *aficionada* of psychoanalysis, "I rather hate therapy altogether—doctors, healers and all the rest. I believe that a real neurotic is a half devil, but a cured neurotic is a perfect devil. . . . I would prefer that neurotics died." In two essays which he wrote about psychoanalysis shortly before his death, Lawrence dismissed it as being too "scientific." Later he called it a fad, and a "mechanistic . . . unconscious illusion."

It is evident that for Lawrence, as well as for Joyce, the lessons of personal experience were more important than the influences of theoretical knowledge. Lawrence's work, as Joyce's does, reflects his own individuality. Lawrence would allow no one either to lead him or think for him. And while he agreed with Freud that sex was the most important thing in the world, he never forgave Freud for "making sex conscious." His mystic strain and his predominantly emotional nature made him despise Freud's painstakingly conscious approach to what Lawrence felt should better be left unconscious. "Adam and Eve fell," Lawrence wrote in a dismissal of psychoanalysis, "not because they had sex . . . but because they *became aware* of their sex and of the possibility of the act." Freud's plea was for the transmutation of the unconscious into the conscious, the rational and the cerebral. Lawrence's plea was the reverse. The non-cerebral were the happiest. Leave well enough alone. The "religion of the blood" was the only true religion. Nevertheless the two men, pleaders as they were for the opposite faces of reality, fought the same battle and trod the same battleground.

Other twentieth-century writers illustrate the same thesis. Kafka's books are deeply "Freudian" not only in the quality and perception of the writing, but in the motives—the escape from his father—which gave them being. But while Kafka's life can be reduced to fairly simple analytic essences, and while his work limns in mystic, ambiguous, irrational fashion the same landscape which Freud depicts in rational, concise fashion, his art is far too complex a construction to be cited simply as an example of direct Freudian influence. Again, both men ploughed the same stony field of modern collapse and sickness. If Freud did not influence Kafka directly, the two men existed in the same spiritual climate, and Kafka, in giving artistic life to Freud's message, as Joyce and Lawrence did, helped to establish in literature the spirit of the Freudian doctrine.

Thomas Mann, who of all modern writers has most explicitly acknowledged his debt to Freud, is as fascinated by death, disease and decay as Freud was. In a sense, *The Magic Mountain* may be said to be the literary counterpart of Freud's scientific formulation of the death instinct. And *Death in Venice*, a portrait of the artist as a neurotic, is again as artistic treatment of a theme which from the beginning concerned the analyst clinically. His *Joseph in Egypt* Mann says he wrote under the inspiration of psychoanalysis, and he calls the book "a union in narrative of psychology and myth which at the same time is a festive meeting of poetry and psychoanalysis." Besides this reflection in his work of a concern with themes which are also those of psychoanalysis, Mann looks optimistically to psychoanalysis as the philosophical and therapeutical salvation for the future. Still, as Hoffmann has summed it up: "It is not that psychoanalysis at some mysterious time changed Mann's views completely around, or even qualified his enthusiasm for them. It is that Mann's interest in a spiritual stocktaking was coincident with his mature acquaintance with psychoanalysis."[102]

Today the popularization of the principles of psychoanalysis continues to spread. Debates rage in the pages of mass circulation magazines over the relative merits of psychoanalysis and religion. In these discussions the ridicule and the scorn that marked the debates of the twenties have for the most part died down. Religion is, of course, still the victor in the majority of battles, but in an increasing number of articles the issue is moot. Almost—if not quite yet—there is seeping into such popular discussions as these the indication that psychoanalysis and religion need not be mutually exclusive; that, in a way, the two can supplement each other.

Side by side with the deepening understanding of psychoanalysis which is reflected in some of the conventional, popular literary work of our present day, there is a stream of experimental, irrational, almost incomprehensible writing, sometimes called surrealist, whose impetus came from the linguistic problem presented by Freud's discovery of the unconscious. At first experimental writers were content with "stream of consciousness" writing, which attempted to reproduce the haphazard flow of the language of the unconscious mind. But writers like Virginia Woolf, Dorothy Richardson and William Faulkner began to expand the frontiers of stream of consciousness in an effort to arrive at an even more plastic representation of the sound and fury of the unconscious mind. From this trend has arisen, not only in writing, but in painting as well, the cult of surrealism, which suspends the laws of ordinary communication on the conscious level and obeys completely the dictates of the unconscious, as the writer feels them. Surrealism in art is the furthest extreme to which Freud's exploration of the unconscious mind has been pushed.

Painting, dancing, the theatre, and music have been influenced by Freud's discoveries just as literature has. Outside the arts the indirect influence of Freud has been equally pervasive. In psychiatry, the principal factors of the psychoanalytic method and philosophy have been quietly assimilated by medical schools which twenty years ago were crying, "Heresy!" and comparing psychoanalysis to phrenology, astrology and alchemy. During the last war, as during the first, the psychoanalytic method received great impetus, and was used in various extensions and applications for the treatment and cure of many psycho-neurotic soldiers. In America, particularly, it has become more and more a part of medicine in so far as it is a therapy, and a part of social science in so far as it deals with human relationships. This interrelation between psychoanalysis and medicine is perhaps best shown in the newly emerging field of psychosomatic medicine, which is concerned with uncovering the influence of psychic factors in producing bodily ills. Today we hear of distinguished physicians estimating that neurotic suffering constitutes fifty to seventy-five per cent of the problems of general medicine.

In the social sciences, the influence of the psychoanalytic point of view has been and continues to be felt. Sociologists like Erich Fromm and John Dollard have been deeply influenced by Freud. Increasingly, sociologists who were formerly intent on pointing out the differences between man's activities as an individual and his activities as a member of society are swinging around to Freud's point of view that social phenomena are in essence an extension of individual attitudes.

Anthropologists like Malinowski and Margaret Mead have also been influenced by Freud. In anthropology, the application of the psychoanalytic method has made for the ready interpretation of heretofore obscure material, and interesting correlations have been drawn between the aspects of the primitive mind as it persists in areas of our civilization and the primitive aspects of the mind as studied by clinical psychoanalysis. In jurisprudence and criminology, as in child psychology, Freud's work is having the growing effect of fostering the substitution of liberal and constructive attitudes for the benighted absolutism and punishing tactics of the era that is passing. Educational methods, following the enlightenment which Freud shed on the child's development, are shifting. As one noted educator, Caroline Zachry, put it: "It has required a tremendously powerful force to turn such a ponderous institution as the school system towards a new direction. That such a force has been at work is apparent in recent trends in education, and the extent to which Freud's discoveries are reflected in these trends is truly impressive—all the more so because this influence upon education is largely indirect. Freud himself did not attempt to formulate the pedagogical implications of psychoanalysis. In all of his writings there are few references to education. It was Anna Freud, a teacher as well as a psychoanalyst, who began the exploration of the indirect application of psychoanalysis to children."[103]

16

Hans im Glueck

The Nazis had burned Freud's books in 1933, in the vain hope that they could destroy the ideas set forth in what they called his "pornographic Jewish speciality." Now, five years later, they had marched into a Vienna not markedly unreceptive to their iron embrace.

Freud had been warned by his friends, family and colleagues all over the world to get out of Austria before the Jew-hating conqueror arrived. Until the Anschluss became a reality, he had said he would leave, but once the Nazis arrived, he hesitated. "Austria is my home," he said, "I must stay." He had lived for forty-two years in the same house in the same street. He had sat at the same desk to write, and in the same chair to read. He had taken all his meals in the dining room with the old-fashioned rosewood furniture. He was eighty-two and the inside of his right jaw was almost entirely eaten away by cancer. He had undergone fifteen operations in so many years, and once every two weeks or so he had had to have his jaw scraped—an ordeal which put him to bed each time for a few days. Pain had become his constant companion, day and night. It is small wonder that he did not think it worth while to uproot himself in order to seek an uneasy sanctuary in a world gone mad for the second time in his life.

But one day in the early spring of 1938 he returned home from having his jaw scraped to find the Gestapo there. The passport and papers which he had obtained in order to enable him to leave on short notice were taken from him. He was forbidden to continue his work. His money was impounded, and the entire stock of books belonging to the publishing house which his son headed was destroyed. The International Psychoanalytical Publishing House was no more. Whatever property he owned was confiscated, and the farm which his daughter Anna owned jointly with Dorothy Burlingham was also taken over by the Reich.

The scientific world feared that Freud himself would be imprisoned. Dr. Ernest Jones flew from London to Vienna to try to persuade Freud to leave. He found Freud still undecided. Finally Jones convinced him—by telling him how an officer of the *Titanic* was brought before a commission of inquiry to explain why he had left the ship instead of going down with it. The officer's reply to his inquisitors had been: "I didn't leave the ship. The ship left me." Freud saw the analogy and agreed at once to leave.

But by this time the Nazis were demanding "ransom." A fund had been raised quietly in American psychoanalytic circles to pay Freud's living expenses after he left Vienna, but the ransom demanded was unexpected and crippling. At this juncture Princess George of Greece, who as Princess Marie Bonaparte had been analysed by Freud, came to the rescue. She offered the Nazis the quarter of a million Austrian schillings she had on deposit in a Vienna bank. The Nazis thought they might do better. Negotiations were prolonged. Meanwhile, William Bullitt, who had also been a patient of Freud's, pulled wires. He asked President Roosevelt to intercede. Roosevelt called the German Ambassador. Finally, the Nazis agreed to let Freud go for the sum the Princess had offered.

Now more delay was in store. Tante Minna had had an operation for a double cataract on her eyes, and had to be in a dark room for two weeks. Finally, early in June 1938, the preparations for departure were complete. The prophet without honour in his own country was prepared at eighty-two to walk in the migratory steps of his people and make his home in a new country. On the eve of his departure he was gay. He had managed to salvage his furniture, some of his books, and the greater part of his collection of ancient *objets d'art*. Standing among the packing-cases, he cried gaily to his nephew—remembering one of the traditional tales of German children—"Now, I'm *Hans im Glueck!*"

On June 4, 1938, Freud—in a wheel chair—Mrs. Freud, Tante Minna, Anna, Dorothy Burlingham, Freud's chow, Lun, and an entourage of patients and servants boarded the Orient Express bound for Paris. In Paris, the party was met by Bullitt and the Princess George, who brought a litter in which to carry Freud off the train. But Freud scorned the litter, and walked, with the aid of a cane, to the waiting car—a fragile death's head dressed jauntily in a green hat and green top-coat. He spent the afternoon resting at Princess George's home, and in the evening the party left for London where Jones had arranged with Sir Samuel Hoare to give Freud permanent sanctuary.

In London at last, where Dr. Jones and Ernst Freud had found a house for the family at Hampstead, near Regent's Park, Freud went immediately to bed. The journey had taxed his feeble strength. To the reporters who immediately stormed the house, Anna was pathetically eager to make it clear that Nazis had treated them well. "Oh, please say how well we were treated," she said. "There were no obstacles. They took our money and some property, but they were polite. I know it is special treatment. Some people are being treated horribly. We are a test case. We came out with full legal rights so that they can point to us as an example of Nazi politeness and freedom to the Jews." During this interview, Martin and Ernst kept up a running cross commentary in German: "Should we say this?" they asked each other. "Had we better say that?" Said Anna: "What we say in the morning will be in Vienna in the evening, and there are others there who are being held. Their treatment depends on us. We are so thankful they let us out."

A steady stream of visitors called at the house—Viennese in exile and British scientists anxious to wish Freud good fortune in his new home. The British Royal Society, which had made him a foreign member in 1936, paid him an almost unprecedented honour by sending its 300-year-old charter books over to him to sign. The Government put an official stamp on his welcome by granting him British nationality.

Soon, with incredible tenacity and endurance, Freud resumed his regular schedule. He rose at eight, was examined by his doctor at ten, and saw a patient before lunch. In the afternoons he wrote—the final draft of *Moses and Monotheism* was completed in about six weeks after his arrival—saw another patient or two, and looked after his correspondence. He left the house rarely, only to go to Harley Street for X-rays, and once or twice to visit Lun, who remained in quarantine for six months.

As Freud's human contacts had dwindled, he had become very fond of dogs. Princess Marie had given him a chow, and Lun, then nine, was one of its offspring. Freud loved and tended Lun devotedly, had her at his side constantly, even during analytic hours. Lun would often tap on the door during a consultation. Freud would let her in and she would lie on the floor and lick herself. "She always behaves psychoanalytically," Freud said. Said the maid: "When the dog doesn't eat, the Herr Professor is unhappy."

The flowers in the garden of the Hampstead house gave him as much pleasure as Lun did. In the rear of the house his architect son, Ernst, had built a loggia facing the garden where Freud spent many hours reclining in a deck chair. When he saw the garden, with its display of lupins, irises and columbines, for the first time, Freud was happy. "I can only say 'Heil Hitler,' " he remarked. Long before that he had explained to a friend the reason for his love of flowers. "Fortunately," he had said, "they have neither character nor complexities."

But soon the cancer which had afflicted him for sixteen years extended beyond the reach of surgical or medical relief. Three weeks after his new country, Great Britain, declared war on Germany—on September 23, 1939—Freud was dead. He was cremated at Golders Green without religious ceremony and his ashes now rest in a twenty-two-hundred-year-old Etruscan vase which he himself brought to London. The vase has been mounted at the top of a tall, slender triangular marble column in the East Columbarium of Golders Green. The inscription on the column is the barest possible statement of fact. It reads: "Sigmund Freud 1856-1939." Like the burial he arranged for his father, his own memorial is simple to a fault.

So he was dead, the man whose unconquerable spirit had battled with the "conqueror worm" for sixteen years. His will to live, despite his "pessimism," despite his "negative philosophy," had been as awesome and terrible as the will to die he had postulated as a psychic truth for all humanity. The worm had lived within him for sixteen years. He had known death in life, intimately. But he had delayed the day of the worm's victory by the strength of his will. He had been more concerned with death than most men, and he had lived longer than most men.

Life for him, he had said repeatedly, had been a duty, a task which as long as his manhood was upon him he was obligated to fulfill. He had died the way he had lived—quietly, resolutely, quite heroically, putting up with the agonizing pain and indignity of his slow death as he had borne the pain of his life. Tobacco had been one of the few indulgences he permitted himself to ease the strain of living. To ease the strain of dying, he consented to an occasional aspirin. Only in the last few hours of his life, when his will to resist "weakness" could no longer function, was any morphine administered. Despite his unalleviated pain and the knowledge that death this time was imminent, despite the sorrow he suffered from the loss and exile of many of his friends, he had, until a few weeks before his death, continued to work.

There were those among the more fanciful of his admirers who had been struck with the symbolic significance of his name: *Sieg* is the German for "victorious" or "victory"; *Mund* is mouth, and thus, by extension, voice or speech. And Sigmund Freud had been truly victorious in speech. His reasoned words had conquered for mankind a domain which had been, until he explored it, a *terra incognita*. But if his mouth had been symbolically the instrument of his victory, it had also been actually the instrument of his defeat. Within his greatest strength lay the seeds of his weakness. For there in his mouth the canker had entered his body. The cancerous evil, the death within life, had chosen the fount of the power and glory of his body to spread its destruction.

This was a bitter joke and an ironic one. Perhaps it was possible for Freud, with his love of bitter jokes, to appreciate this final irony. But it is unlikely that he would have been content to ascribe the cause of his death to accident—just as he had never been content to ascribe the causes or motivations of his life to accident. He might very well have cast his mind back to those constitutional facts of his life which had contributed fatefully, intricately, to the deliberate design of his death.

As a child of two or three, he had climbed on a footstool in the pantry of the Freiberg house, in order to reach a sweet resting high on a chest. Under his unsure footing, the footstool collapsed and its edge struck him forcibly behind his lower jaw. He was badly hurt. There is reason to believe that the injury he sustained then was just such an "infective lesion" as he once described psychoanalysis as being. For the cancer struck the area of the jaw he had injured as a child.

His mouth was the only area of his body he would allow himself to indulge and pamper. Smoking was his one "vice," his one weakness. And the first signs of irritation in his mouth were caused by excessive smoking. Although he was warned, the smoking continued and the irritation grew into a cancer. Such excessive, virtually compulsive smoking as Freud's has always been interpreted psychoanalytically, since Freud's first formulations of character types, as evidence of a strong oral impulse. That Freud, weighed on the scales of his own theories, was an "oral type" is indisputable. Not only the smoking, which in his case lit the fuse that destroyed him, but other characteristics and impulses which he ascribed to those people who remained fixed at this pregenital phase of maturing, were his. He had enumerated among strong "oral" characteristics, ambition, envy and a tendency to self-punishment. These were prominent among his own character traits.

In the end, Freud defeated himself. After a life longer and more fruitful than those achieved by ordinary men, he went to his death bitter, unhappy and convinced of failure. He had explored and charted a new universe, but he had neither succeeded in solving the riddle of himself nor, for all the brilliance and profundity of the answers he dredged up, the riddle of the universe. He had, like David, who was also marked out by destiny, used a slingshot to conquer the giant opposed to the forces of righteousness. Freud's slingshot—the limited, archaic tool of reason—had assured a partial victory. It had confounded and defeated the Philistines, but it had not brought the victor the full enjoyment of victory.

Freud, whether constitutionally or environmentally, whether innately or circumstantially, had been an insatiable man. He had believed himself capable of understanding everything. A pitiless disillusionist, he had cherished, with the exaggerated absolutism that was spine to his rigidity, a single illusion: knowledge is power. He had tried his best for full knowledge. He had looked at life with the cold, ironic, disillusioned eye of Death itself. He had dared to psychoanalyse God. He had resolutely—and it took great courage—stripped life bare of golden mist, rosy illusion, and the pleasurable haze of wishful thinking. He had, in the doing, enlarged and corrected man's astigmatic vision of the universe which is himself. If each man, after Freud's discoveries, still remained an island, he remained an island linked to his brothers by a chain of communication undreamed of before Freud's time.

But the cold cables which link the islands—banishers of loneliness and isolation though they are—provide neither the comfort nor the solace that their discoverer, no less than other men, needed. The light which Freud shed on the problems of mankind was a biting, cold north light. There was neither peace in it nor mercy. And while it brightened recesses of the human spirit that had been dark and frightening, the light was not consoling.

Freud pinned his faith to this intellectual light. But in

its harsh severity he could find no nourishment for the hunger of his soul. He had sought truth, and would not accept it on faith. He found a larger share of truth than all but one or two men of his time. He revealed humanity to itself, but he could not make it any happier than he could make himself. For without all the answers, he was required to accept something on faith—a faith somewhat different from that which had permeated religion. By the question of faith he had been obsessed. He had dissected and analysed it in all his studies of the religious impulse, until there remained for him no warm tissue to clothe its stripped bones. So, he rejected the faith of his fathers, and clung instead to a faith in the power of reason.

As his life spent itself out, he saw himself that this kind of faith was not enough. But he had lived side by side with the probing scalpel and the microscope too long to exchange them for the altar cloth and the Covenant of the Ark. No theologian had ever fought more fervently for the dignity and survival of the human soul. No man had been at bottom a greater humanist. And no humanist had, in the end, been less human.

He had found the real world hard and unreasonable. But the eminently reasonable world he created in order to understand it eluded his understanding finally no less than the real world. He had made only one basic mistake: he had believed that everything could be understood. He had insisted that the limited world of reason and reasonable actions was the one reality. No less rigidly than the Spartans, the Biblical Jews, the Calvinists and the Puritans, he had built a monistic world, in which only one solution was possible and one path visible. He had chipped away at himself, this sculptor of his own spirit: here he chiselled off the will to pleasure, there he carved away the need to relax and relent. Out went the faith in a shower of marble dust. Off came the emotion, the feeling, the impulsive actions, the wishes and the fantasies.

The statue of himself he chiselled was an heroic one. He emerged at last as one of the supreme intellectual heroes of our time, and every sentence he wrote is bathed with the heroism of his effort to see and understand everything.

But for this *tour de force* he paid the penalty of his humanity. In the end, as a human being, and not as an agent of destiny, he resembled nothing so much as the rigid, immobile marble giant with whom he had first fallen in love in 1913 in the Corso Cavour. It never profited Sigmund Freud that he had gained a whole new world, for, although he never lost his soul, he would never admit that he could find it.

Sources and Acknowledgments

1. *The Interpretation of Dreams,* by Sigmund Freud. The Macmillan Co.
2. *The Basic Writings of Sigmund Freud,* by Sigmund Freud. Random House.
3. *The Interpretation of Dreams,* by Sigmund Freud. The Macmillan Co.
4. Ibid.
5. *Vienna,* by H. D. Sedgwick. The Bobbs-Merrill Co.
6. *Freud, Master and Friend,* by Hanns Sachs. Harvard University Press.
7. Ibid.
8. *Vienna,* by H. D. Sedgwick. The Bobbs-Merrill Company.
9. *The Interpretation of Dreams,* by Sigmund Freud. The Macmillan Co.
10. Ibid.
11. Ibid.
12. Ibid.
13. *Psychopathology of Everyday Life,* by Sigmund Freud. The Macmillan Co.
14. *Sigmund Freud,* by Fritz Wittels. Allen & Unwin, Ltd.
15. *The Interpretation of Dreams,* by Sigmund Freud. The Macmillan Co.
16. *Autobiography,* by Sigmund Freud. W. W. Norton & Co.
17. *History of the Psychoanalytic Movement,* by Sigmund Freud. The Nervous and Mental Disease Publishing Co.
18. Ibid.

19. Ibid.
20. *Stuedien uber Hysterie*, by Breuer and Freud. F. Deuticke, Leipzig and Vienna.
21. *Autobiography*, by Sigmund Freud. W. W. Norton & Co.
22. *The Interpretation of Dreams*, by Sigmund Freud. The Macmillan Co.
23. Ibid.
24. *Psychopathology of Everyday Life*, by Sigmund Freud. The Macmillan Co.
25. *The Interpretation of Dreams*, by Sigmund Freud. The Macmillan Co.
26. *History of the Psychoanalytic Movement*, by Sigmund Freud. The Nervous and Mental Disease Publishing Co.
27. *The Interpretation of Dreams*, by Sigmund Freud. The Macmillan Co.
28. *History of the Psychoanalytic Movement*, by Sigmund Freud. The Nervous and Mental Disease Publishing Co.
29. Ibid.
30. *Freud, Master and Friend*, by Hanns Sachs. Harvard University Press.
31. *Psychopathology of Everyday Life*, by Sigmund Freud. The Macmillan Co.
32. "Reminiscences of Freud," by Max Graf. *Psychoanalytic Quarterly*, 1942.
33. *History of the Psychoanalytic Movement*, by Sigmund Freud. The Nervous and Mental Disease Publishing Co.
34. *Freud, Master and Friend*, by Hanns Sachs. Harvard University Press.
35. *Sigmund Freud*, by Fritz Wittels. Allen & Unwin, Ltd.
36. *Introduction to the Basic Writings of Sigmund Freud*, by A. A. Brill, Random House.
37. "Fragments of a Freudian Analysis," by Joseph Wortis, *American Journal of Orthopsychiatry*, Vol. X, No. 4, October 1940.
38. *Sigmund Freud*, by Fritz Wittels. Allen & Unwin, Ltd.
39. *On Being of the B'nai B'rith*, by Sigmund Freud. Commentary.
40. Ibid.
41. "Jung and National Socialism", by Feldman, *American Journal of Psychiatry*, September 1945.
42. *History of the Psychoanalytic Movement*, by Sigmund Freud. The Nervous and Mental Disease Publishing Co.
43. *Sigmund Freud*, by Fritz Wittels. Allen & Unwin, Ltd.

44. "Fragments of a Freudian Analysis," by Joseph Wortis, *American Journal of Orthopsychiatry*, Vol. X, No. 4, October 1940.
45. *History of the Psychoanalytic Movement*, by Sigmund Freud. The Nervous and Mental Disease Publishing Co.
46. Ibid.
47. "Writing on the Wall," by H. D., *Life and Letters Today*, 1945.
48. *Psychopathology of Everyday Life*, by Sigmund Freud. The Macmillan Co.
49. Ibid.
50. Ibid.
51. "Reminiscences of Freud," by Max Graf. *Psychoanalytic Quarterly*, 1942.
52. *Mind, Medicine and Man*, Gregory Zilboorg. Harcourt, Brace & Co.
53. *Autobiography*, by Sigmund Freud. W. W. Norton & Co.
54. Ibid.
54a. *Glimpses of the Great*, by S. Viereck. The Macaulay Co.
54b. *Men of Turmoil*, chapter by J. L. Grey. Minton-Balch Co.
55. *The Collected Works of Sigmund Freud*, Vol. IV, by Sigmund Freud. The Hogarth Press.
55a. Ibid.
56. *The Interpretation of Dreams*, by Sigmund Freud. The Macmillan Co.
57. *Leonardo da Vinci*, by Sigmund Freud. Random House.
58. *Freud and His Times*, by Fritz Wittels. Liveright Publishing Corp.
59. *Leonardo da Vinci*, by Sigmund Freud. Random House.
60. *The Collected Works of Sigmund Freud*, Vol. IV, by Sigmund Freud. The Hogarth Press.
61. *Leonardo da Vinci*, by Sigmund Freud. Random House.
61a. Ibid.
62. Ibid.
63. *Autobiography*, by Sigmund Freud. W. W. Norton & Co.
64. *The Interpretation of Dreams*, by Sigmund Freud. The Macmillan Co.
65. "The Dreams Freud Dreamed," by Immanual Velikovsky. *Psychoanalytic Review*, 1941.

66. "Regarding Freud's Book on Moses," by Oehlschlegel. *Psychoanalytic Review*, 1943.
67. *The Collected Works of Sigmund Freud*, Vol. IV, by Sigmund Freud. The Hogarth Press.
68. Ibid.
69. Ibid.
70. "Regarding Freud's Book on Moses," by Oehlschlegel. *Psychoanalytic Review*, 1943.
71. *Freud, Master and Friend*, by Hanns Sachs. Harvard University Press.
72. Ibid.
73. *Psychopathology of Everyday Life*, by Sigmund Freud. The Macmillan Co.
74. Ibid.
75. "Writing on the Wall," by H. D. *Life and Letters Today*, 1945.
76. "Fragments of a Freudian Analysis," by Joseph Wortis, *American Journal of Orthopsychiatry*, Vol. X, No. 4, October 1940.
77. "Reminiscences of a Personal Contact with Freud," by Roy Grinker. *American Journal of Orthopsychiatry*, Vol X, No. 4, October 1940.
78. "Writing on the Wall," by H. D. *Life and Letters Today*, 1945.
80. "Obituary of Freud," by Ernest Jones. *International Journal of Psychoanalysis*, 1940.
81. *The Collected Works of Sigmund Freud*, Vol. IV, by Sigmund Freud. The Hogarth Press.
82. *Three Contributions to the Theory of Sex*, by Sigmund Freud, Random House.
83. *New Introductory Lectures on Psychoanalysis, by* Sigmund Freud. W. W. Norton & Co.
84. Ibid.
85. *The Collected Works of Sigmund Freud*, Vol. IV, by Sigmund Freud. The Hogarth Press.
86. "Fragments of a Freudian Analysis," by Joseph Wortis. *American Journal of Orthopsychiatry*, Vol. X, No. 4, October, 1940.
87. *Psychopathology of Everyday Life*, by Sigmund Freud. The Macmillan Co.
88. *The Collected Works of Sigmund Freud*, Vol. IV, by Sigmund Freud. The Hogarth Press.
89. *Mental Healers*, by Stefan Zweig. The Viking Press.

90. *Autobiography*, by Sigmund Freud. W. W. Norton & Co.
91. Ibid.
92. *Mental Healers*, by Stefan Zweig. The Viking Press.
93. *In the American Jungle*, by Waldo Frank. Farrar, Rinehart, Inc.
94. *Men of Turmoil*, chapter by J. L. Grey. Minton-Balch Co.
95. *The Future of an Illusion*, by Sigmund Freud. The Hogarth Press.
96. Ibid.
98. Ibid.
97. Ibid.
99. *The Collected Works of Sigmund Freud*, Vol. IV, by Sigmund Freud. The Hogarth Press.
100. *Movers and Shakers*, by Mabel Dodge Luhan. Harcourt, Brace & Co.
101. "Dreiser on Freud," by Theodore Dreiser. *Psychoanalytic Review*, July 1931.
102. *Freudianism and the Literary Mind*, by Frederick J. Hoffman. Louisiana State University Press.
103. Article by Caroline Zachry. *Psychoanalytic Quarterly*, 1941.